Introduction to Animal Technology

Second Edition

Revised by

Stephen W. Barnett
Technical Education Consultant
Formerly Senior Lecturer
City of Westminster College
Vice President of the Institute of Animal Technology

Published for
The Institute of Animal Technology

First edition published as Principles of Animal Technology I
edited by *P J Kelly, K G Millican and Pam Organ*

Blackwell
Science

© 2001
by Blackwell Science Ltd
Editorial Offices:
Osney Mead, Oxford OX2 0EL
25 John Street, London WC1N 2BS
23 Ainslie Place, Edinburgh EH3 6AJ
350 Main Street, Malden
    MA 02148 5018, USA
54 University Street, Carlton
    Victoria 3053, Australia
10, rue Casimir Delavigne
    75006 Paris, France

Other Editorial Offices:

Blackwell Wissenschafts-Verlag GmbH
Kurfürstendamm 57
10707 Berlin, Germany

Blackwell Science KK
MG Kodenmacho Building
7-10 Kodenmacho Nihombashi
Chuo-ku, Tokyo 104, Japan

Iowa State University Press
A Blackwell Science Company
2121 S. State Avenue
Ames, Iowa 50014-8300, USA

First published 1988 by The Institute of Animal
Technology under the title *The Principles of Animal
Technology I*
Reprinted 1992
Second edition published by Blackwell Science Ltd,
2001 under the title *Introduction to Animal Technology*

Set in 10 on 12pt Times
by Best-set Typesetter Ltd., Hong Kong
Printed and bound in Great Britain by
MPG Books, Bodmin, Cornwall

DISTRIBUTORS

Marston Book Services Ltd
PO Box 269
Abingdon
Oxon OX14 4YN
(*Orders*: Tel: 01235 465500
            Fax: 01235 465555)

USA and Canada
    Iowa State University Press
    A Blackwell Science Company
    2121 S. State Avenue
    Ames, Iowa 50014-8300
    (*Orders:* Tel: 800-862-6657
               Fax: 515-292-3348
               Web   www.isupress.com
               email: orders@isupress.com)

Australia
    Blackwell Science Pty Ltd
    54 University Street
    Carlton, Victoria 3053
    (*Orders:* Tel: 03 9347 0300
               Fax: 03 9347 5001)

A catalogue record for this title
is available from the British Library

ISBN 0-632-05594-4

Library of Congress
Cataloging-in-Publication Data
is available

For further information on
Blackwell Science, visit our website:
www.blackwell-science.com

Contents

Preface

The first edition of this book was published by the Institute of Animal Technology (IAT) under the title *Principles of Animal Technology 1*. The editors, John Kelly, Keith Millican and Pam Organ, produced a book that has proved to be a valuable resource for technicians beginning a career in animal technology.

Although the basic principles of animal technology remain constant there have been some important developments since this book first appeared and these have led to the need for this revised edition. As an example, significant change has been caused by the Animals (Scientific Procedures) Act 1986. In the 12 year life of *Principles of Animal Technology 1*, several Codes of Practice and a new schedule (2A) have been introduced and two existing schedules (1 and 2) have been amended. These have all had some effect on the way animals are kept and used in animal facilities.

Like the first edition, the contents of this book closely follow the syllabuses for the animal technology unit of the IAT Certificate examination and the Animal Technology unit of the BTEC First Certificate in Science (Animal Technology). A chapter on animal house safety has been added to reflect changes in the IAT Certificate syllabus.

The publication of this book has been supported by the Institute of Animal Technology as part of its aim to ensure the welfare of animals bred and used for scientific procedures by the promotion of education and training. The Institute also produces four video tapes, *Handle with Care*, *Procedures with Care*, *Euthanasia with Care* and *Routine Care*, which are relevant to the subjects covered in this book. Information on the work of the Institute can be obtained from the website http://iat.org.uk.

The well-being of laboratory animals relies to a great extent on animal technicians carrying out their work knowledgeably and conscientiously. It is to be hoped that this edition of *An Introduction to Animal Technology* will be as helpful to technicians in fulfilling their role as the first edition was.

Acknowledgements

I must acknowledge that this is not an original work; the editors and contributors of the first edition of the book produced an excellent text to revise.

I would like to record my thanks to the people who have helped with the preparation of this revision. Jas Barley, Roger Francis, Brian Lowe and Sarah Lane read the manuscript and made many useful suggestions. I have also tried out chapters of the book on many of my students and have noted their comments. I am grateful for the time and trouble that all of these people have taken to read and comment on the text. Of course if any mistakes remain they are my responsibility.

Roger Francis allowed me to disrupt his unit on many occasions so that I could take photographs. Jas Barley and others also let me into their units to take photographs. I am grateful to all of them.

Martin Heath of GlaxoSmithKline plc organised many of the illustrations to be taken. I am grateful to him for saving me a great deal of work.

I am grateful to the following people and organisations for giving me permission to use their illustrations: A. Buckwell (Figs 1.4, 1.5), CBD, DERA (Fig. 10.10), Prof P. A. Flecknell (Figs 1.3, 1.4, 1.6, 11.2, 11.3, Plate 8), Lillico Biotechnology (Fig. 5.1), Dr T. Morris, GSK (Fig. 2.9) and Rentokil Initial (Figs 7.9–11, 7.14b, 7.15).

Contributors

CONTRIBUTORS TO FIRST EDITION

Editors

P. J. Kelly, K. G. Millican, Pamela J. Organ

Contributors

T. D. Hornett, Georgina L. Owen, G. C. Bantin

CONTRIBUTORS TO SECOND EDITION

P. J. Kelly, Trish Hayes, G. Childs, R. J. Francis.

Chapter 1
Animal Health

The production and maintenance of healthy animals is a primary function of animal technicians. The cleaning routines, hygiene measures, environmental controls and provision of adequate diets, discussed later in this book, all contribute to ensuring laboratory animals stay free of disease.

Disease can be defined as any condition that interferes with the well-being of an animal; it can be infectious or non-infectious. Infectious diseases are caused by specific organisms (e.g. bacteria, viruses, fungi or invertebrate parasites) and are passed from one animal to another by direct (contact) or indirect means (in the air, on food etc.).

All other causes of disease are non-infectious. Examples of non-infectious diseases include physical injury (wounds from fighting), inherited abnormalities (tooth malocclusion), nutritional imbalance (vitamin C deficiency in guinea pigs), inappropriate environment (ringtail in rats), absorption of toxic substances and stress. Stress can occur whenever the internal environment of an animal is upset. If the upset is short term and relatively minor the animal's homeostatic mechanism will return it to balance quickly but if the upset is prolonged or extreme this may not happen and the animal will show signs of stress. Stress will accompany all of the types of disease mentioned above or can be brought about by environmental pressures (e.g. overcrowding, bullying), or as the result of experimental procedures.

Disease in an animal colony results in the suffering of individual animals; if the disease is infectious the whole colony could be affected. Whatever the cause of the disease, breeding performance and experimental results will be compromised. Sick animals do not make good experimental models because the physiological changes in their bodies caused by the disease will alter the way in which they respond to experimental procedures. Similarly sick animals do not breed well; if they produce any young at all the young will be weak and sickly themselves.

Therefore it is essential to take every precaution to keep disease out of the animal unit and to ensure that if any animal is in poor health it is identified at the earliest possible moment to prevent suffering, reduce the risk of spread and prevent invalidating experimental results.

ASSESSMENT OF HEALTH STATUS

In order to detect signs of disease in an animal it is necessary to have knowledge of its normal appearance and behaviour. This is gained by observing animals in their cages and when they are being cleaned or handled. Any divergence from the norm could indicate disease and the animal should be more closely inspected.

Monitoring health status is a continuous process. Every time a cage is passed, every time an animal is removed from its cage and every time it is fed or watered, it should be observed for signs of ill health (Fig. 1.1).

Factors that should be observed include:

Movement	Abnormal gait, lack of movement.
Posture	Hunched, head or limb held at odd angle.

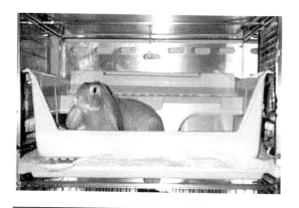

Fig. 1.1 Healthy, alert rabbit in its cage.

Isolation	Separation from other animals in the cage, coat condition, hair rough and erect (staring coat), lack of grooming.
Food	Ignored, mouthed (food taken into the mouth then dropped so it is wet), excessive intake.
Water	Ignored or excessive intake.
Temperament	Signs of apprehension and aggression in an otherwise friendly animal.
Faeces and urine	Too much, too little or abnormal (e.g. containing blood).
Discharges	Haemorrhage, mucus, vomit (in animals that can vomit; mice, rats, Syrian hamsters, guinea pigs and rabbits cannot).
Weight	Unexpected gain or loss.
Respiration	Rate abnormal or noisy.

Detailed health inspections

In addition to the constant observation described above, it is necessary to carry out more thorough inspections of individual animals and most animal house routines incorporate detailed examinations on a regular basis. Routine examinations are necessary in breeding colonies when selecting future breeding stock, when weaning and when selecting animals for culling. Health assessments are also necessary when selecting animals for experimental use.

When performing a detailed health check it is necessary to follow a routine so that no point is overlooked. Observations of the cage and the animal whilst it is moving are as important as physically examining the animal. Any signs of ill health that are revealed during the inspection, however trivial, should be reported to a senior member of staff without delay.

Examination of a rabbit for signs of ill health

The principles of a detailed health examination are the same for all species although the different species may suffer from different diseases. The rabbit makes a good model to learn from because of its size.

The examination starts by watching the animal at rest in its cage. Normal breathing is rather rapid (30–60 breaths per minute) and shallow compared to the human. A change in rate or depth of respiration could indicate a respiratory infection. The rabbit should be quiet and relaxed. Following removal of the rabbit, the cage should be inspected to assess:

- The amount (too much or too little) of food and water consumed.
- The amount, colour, form, smell and consistency of faeces.
- The amount, colour and smell of urine.
- The presence of mucus or blood.

Close inspection of the rabbit should be made on a flat, non-slip surface so that it feels secure (Fig. 1.2). The inspection should follow a logical sequence beginning with the mouth, working along the back and then underneath to the forepaws.

The mouth

Normal appearance	The mouth should have a clean appearance, the lips, gums and tongue should have a pink colour.
Possible abnormalities	Lesions (sores, cuts);

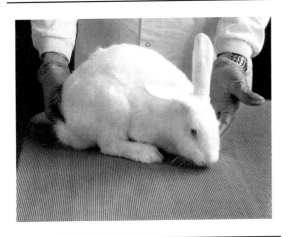

Fig. 1.2 Rabbit placed on a non-slip surface for health assessment.

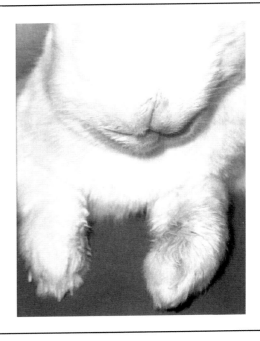

Fig. 1.3 Rabbit with 'snuffles'. Note discharge around the nose and matted fur on fore paws.

inflammation (redness, swelling and heat); mis-aligned (malocclusion), overgrown or broken teeth.

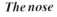

The nose

Normal appearance	The nostrils and surrounding fur should be clean and dry.
Possible abnormalities	Signs of matted fur, wetness or discharge indicating a respiratory disorder such as snuffles. There may also be abnormal respiratory sounds, e.g. rattling, gurgling and wheezing. Matted fur on the inside of the forelegs may also indicate respiratory disease as the rabbit wipes its nose with its paws (Fig. 1.3).

The eyes and eyelids

Normal appearance	The eyelids should be clean and the eyes clear and bright.
Possible abnormalities	The lids may be swollen or inflamed, encrusted, stuck with mucus or weeping with a watery discharge. The cornea may be opaque (cloudy) or the sclera (the white of the eye) may be discoloured or inflamed. If only one eye is affected the cause may be a foreign body. If both eyes are affected it is more likely to be an infection.

The ears

Normal appearance	Each earflap (pinna) should be well furred on the outside and clean on

the inside right down into the meatus (ear canal). It should feel warm.

Possible abnormalities — Lack of fur may indicate scratching due to irritation in the ear. A yellow/brown crust deep in the inside of the pinna may indicate ear canker, a condition caused by the mite *Psorptes cuniculi*.

The body, coat, back and sides

Hands are passed gently along the back and sides of the rabbit to check for lumps and bumps (abscesses, cysts and wounds). The spine should feel knobbly in the lumbar region and well muscled on either side. Any evidence of weight loss will be apparent in this region and could be due to several factors, e.g. malnutrition, dehydration and old age. The coat should be sleek and shiny. Although rabbits lose some fur continuously and may have periods of heavy moult, a good under fur should remain, and there should be no bald patches. The loose skin on the back should be pinched up and allowed to fall (tenting). The speed at which it returns to normal gives an indication of the state of hydration. If it takes a long time the animal may be dehydrated.

The tail and anus

The tail and anus should be clean without evidence of adhered faeces or mucus and have no signs of inflammation or prolapsed rectum.

The genitalia

Females – The normal appearance can vary considerably depending on the stage of oestrous cycle. In oestrus the vulva is swollen and inflamed. Any bloody or purulent (pus-like) discharge could indicate infection.
Males – Sexually mature males should have two well-developed testes. Occasionally one or both testes do not descend into the scrotum. Injury to testes may result from keeping males together.

The penis should not show any signs of abnormal discharge.

The hind legs

The hind legs should be checked for swollen, damaged or stiff joints and sore hocks.

The feet should be checked for broken, torn or overgrown claws.

The abdomen, thorax and axillae

The fur is naturally thinner in these regions, which aids inspection of the skin. Evidence of ectoparasites, e.g. scratches, inflammation, baldness and scurf, may be more apparent. It may also be possible to see parasites, their eggs and faeces.

It is normal for a late-pregnant, pseudo pregnant or lactating doe to strip the fur from her underbelly, so fur loss in these animals is not normally a cause of concern. Does may strip their fur at other times. The mammary glands should be checked for number and position of teats (eight is usual in the rabbit), and palpable lumps which could be caused by tumours or infections (mastitis).

The fore legs

The length of the claws should be checked and the inside of the fore legs for evidence of nasal discharge.

The chin

Soreness or wetness may be present, caused by problems in the mouth.

General

Some rabbits develop a habit of rubbing themselves on their food hoppers or water bottle spouts, which may give rise to sores particularly in the head and neck region. The rabbit should be observed at rest and in movement for alertness and awareness of its surroundings, for free and easy movements and normal gait and posture. Any abnormalities could indicate damage to the spine or limbs, which is not otherwise obvious. Rabbits are particularly prone to back injuries.

Handling for health inspection

The above checks involve handling the rabbit and suitable techniques need to be learned with advice from an experienced person.

AMELIORATION OF CONDITIONS FOUND ON HEALTH INSPECTIONS

Amelioration means to improve or make better. If routine observations or detailed health checks of an animal disclose conditions that give cause for concern, experienced colleagues should be informed immediately. Some examples of improving the condition of animals with specific conditions are given below but it should be emphasised that all deviations from the normal condition of an animal must be reported to the appropriate person and must be recorded according to local rules.

Overgrown teeth

This abnormality may start with one or more teeth being broken and, as the incisors of rabbits and rodents continually grow, the teeth are unable to wear themselves down on the corresponding missing tooth. Alternatively the cause may be due to malocclusion (failure of incisor teeth to meet) which is an inherited trait and animals with this condition should not be used for breeding (Figs 1.4, 1.5).

Cases of overgrown or broken teeth should be reported to a person competent to trim the teeth. If the cause of overgrowth is malocclusion the condition will return so the animals need to be regularly inspected and the treatment repeated.

Sore hocks

Sore hocks were common when rabbits were housed on grid floors. The uneven grid resulted in the weight of the rabbit being unevenly distributed over the foot; it was borne on local areas

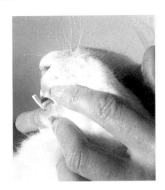

Fig. 1.4 Overgrown rabbit teeth.

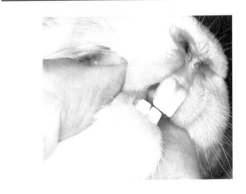

Fig. 1.5 Normal rabbit teeth.

corresponding to the high point of the grids. The situation is aggravated by poor hygiene and obesity.

The condition is similar to pressure sores in humans. The pressure causes irritation, hair loss and thickening of the skin, which eventually breaks and becomes ulcerated. The wounds provide a route for infectious organisms to enter the body and affect internal organs (Fig. 1.6).

Fortunately with the increased use of perforated floors rather than grids the condition is much less common. If it does occur, the rabbit should be kept on a solid floor and given clean sawdust and sterilised hay as bedding.

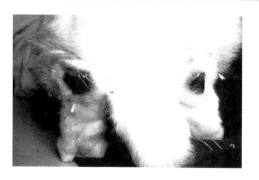

Fig. 1.6 Sore hocks in rabbit.

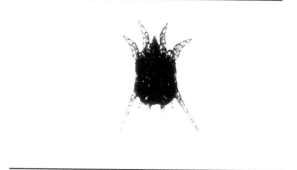

Fig. 1.8 Ear canker mite.

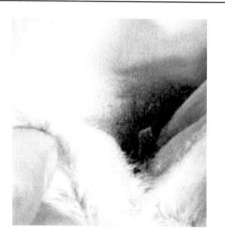

Fig. 1.7 Ear canker.

Ear canker

The ear canker mite *Psorptes cuniculi* lives on the surface of the skin, punctures it and feeds off the tissue fluid that leaks from the puncture wounds. The tissue fluid forms a yellow/brown crust under which the mites can be found (Figs 1.7, 1.8). The crust can be removed and examined microscopically for mites, their cast-off skin and faeces to confirm the cause of the condition. The mites cause intense irritation to the rabbit which may scratch continually at its ears. Fortunately the condition is now very rare in laboratory animal units and where it is found is readily treated. The best treatments are prescription only medicines (POM) which can be obtained on the advice of the named veterinary surgeon.

Overgrown claws

Rabbits need their claws clipped regularly. Overgrown claws are painful and affect the way an animal walks. If they are allowed to overgrow for too long it becomes impossible to trim them back to their correct length.

Clipping is a straightforward process; a pair of clippers is all that is required. The animal must be firmly restrained because, although the procedure is not painful if carried out properly, rabbits object to it (Figs 1.9, 1.10). It is necessary to be aware of the blood vessels and nerves (often called the 'quick') that run down the centre of the claw. The longer the claw grows the further down the claw they grow. In light coloured animals the quick can be seen, in dark animals it cannot. To avoid damaging the quick it is best to clip the claws little and often.

PAIN

Pain often accompanies disease but may occur

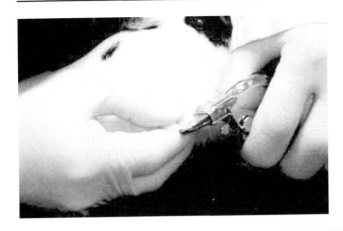

Fig. 1.9 Clipping rabbit claw.

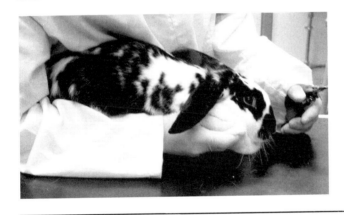

Fig. 1.10 Restraining rabbits to clip claws.

where there are no obvious signs of ill health. It is therefore important to recognise signs that indicate an animal is in pain:

- *Appearance* – Animals in pain often isolate themselves from cage mates and sit hunched in the corner of their cage. They may not groom so the coat becomes scruffy and there may be soiling around the anus. Mostly they are immobile but when they move they may have an abnormal gait.
- *Food and water intake* – There is a marked reduction in food and water intake which, in single housed animals, should be noticeable by the amount of food left in the hopper and water in the bottle. There will be a consequential loss of body mass and lower amount of faeces and urine produced.
- *Temperament* – Animals that are usually easy to handle may become aggressive, particularly when the area that is causing pain is approached.
- *Vocalisation* – The amount of sound produced by an animal in pain differs with species and the degree of pain being experienced. Few animals make a noise all the time although dogs may whine for long periods. Animals in pain may cry out when being handled; in some cases these

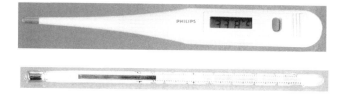

Fig. 1.11 Electronic and mercury thermometers.

cries may be in ultra sound which cannot be perceived by humans.

Interpreting some of the signs of pain can be difficult for an inexperienced person. Wherever there is doubt more experienced colleagues should be consulted.

BODY TEMPERATURE

Further evidence of the physiological condition of an animal may be obtained by measuring the body temperature. A variation in the body temperature of an endothermic (homeothermic) animal of 1 or 2 degrees Celsius (°C) could indicate ill health.

The body temperature of a rabbit is measured by inserting a thermometer into its rectum. Two main types of thermometer are used: the mercury in glass clinical thermometer and electronic thermometers using thermocouple or semi-conductor probes (Fig. 1.11).

In either case the thermometer or the probe should be clean and disinfected with a suitable agent such as 70% alcohol.

Measuring the body temperature of a rabbit

The rabbit is removed from its cage taking care not to excite it, as this will affect the body temperature. It must be restrained by a suitable method, for instance in stocks, wrapped in a towel or by a second person holding it.

Technique using a mercury in glass thermometer

Before inserting the thermometer into the rectum it has to be checked to ensure that the mercury level is below the starting point of the scale. If it is

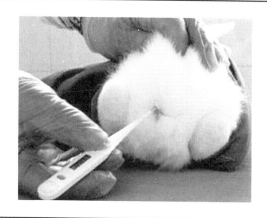

Fig. 1.12 Taking the rectal temperature of a rabbit.

not, the mercury is shaken down by holding the top of the instrument and flicking the wrist.

The thermometer should be lubricated with Vaseline or other lubricating jelly and gently inserted into the rectum whilst holding the tail out of the way (Fig. 1.12). Rotating it may ease the insertion. Force must not be used; resistance to insertion may be caused by a faecal pellet or by the rectal wall and slight alteration of the angle of insertion should avoid the problem.

The thermometer should be inserted so that the bulb is completely enclosed by the rectum and is in contact with the rectal wall. It should be held in position for the time stated on it or in the instructions accompanying it (usually 0.5 to 2 minutes). Immediately it is removed, the temperature should be read and noted. If the mercury column is not easily visible the thermometer can be slowly rotated until it comes into view.

After the animal has been returned to its cage

the thermometer should be cleaned, disinfected, shaken down and safely stored so that it is ready for use.

Using an electronic thermometer

Electronic thermometers are becoming more popular than mercury in glass instruments. They have the advantage of presenting the temperature in a digital form, which removes possible human error from reading the instrument. They also eliminate the danger of exposure to broken glass and mercury if the fragile thermometer is broken.

An electronic thermometer is used in the same way as a mercury in glass instrument but instead of zeroing the mercury the battery must be checked to ensure it will give an accurate reading.

Temperature range

As soon as the temperature is recorded the rabbit should be returned to its cage. The temperature obtained from a healthy rabbit should be within 1°C of 39.5°C. Pregnant does or does in oestrus may exhibit greater variation.

Chapter 2
Caging and Housing

Laboratory animals spend almost all of their lives within a cage or pen; it is therefore essential that, as far as possible, their accommodation provides for all of their needs.

Cages should incorporate the following essential features:

- The safe containment of the animal.
- Provision of the animal's needs to enable it to fulfil as wide a range of its natural behaviour as possible. This means enough space for exercise, defaecating, urinating, grooming, social activity, privacy and where appropriate giving birth and rearing young. The cage must also allow adequate light and fresh air and an appropriate temperature and humidity to reach the occupants.
- Be easy to use and service. The cage should be easy to clean, to provide food and water and to get the animal into and out of safely. The animal should be able to be seen easily.
- Be economic in use. Cages must be able to withstand the attention of their occupants and the cleaning routines (cage wash, autoclave, disinfectants) they will be exposed to. Economic considerations involve a balance of the initial cost and the length of time they can be used.
- Comply with experimental needs.

The design of a cage is always a compromise between these factors and, where a compromise cannot be reached, cages that are designed for specific purposes have to be used. For instance if a 24 hour urine collection is required from a rodent it would be necessary to use a metabolism cage (see Chapter 11).

A wide range of cages are available 'off the shelf' from specialist manufacturers who will also build animal accommodation to specific design (see Table 2.1).

CAGING MATERIALS

A variety of materials are used to manufacture cages and pens for laboratory animals. Consideration of the physical properties of these materials helps to assess their usefulness for particular purposes:

- *Strength* – rigidity and ability to resist animal activity and normal wear and tear in the animal unit. Metals are very strong. Stainless steel or galvanised mild steel are suitable for large animal accommodation. Plastics are less strong and are suitable to house rodents.
- *Density* – defined as its mass per unit volume. It is a useful measure to compare the heaviness of objects of different shapes. Metals are much more dense than plastics.
- *Thermal conductivity* – the ability of a material to conduct heat. Metals are good conductors and therefore conduct heat rapidly. Plastics and wood are poor conductors; poor conductors are good insulators. Where temperatures vary greatly thermal conductivity is of great importance.

If a rabbit was housed in a metal hutch outdoors in the winter, it would probably die of hypothermia because the metal would conduct

Table 2.1 Some features of cage design.

Feature	Advantages	Disadvantages
Solid floor	Prevents up-draughts, allows nest building, fewer injuries, especially to young	Limits ventilation, bedding/nesting materials need frequent changing as they become soiled
Mesh or perforated floor	Needs less frequent, less arduous cleaning, allows better ventilation	Cannot be used for breeding small species, allows draughts, can cause injuries if not exactly right for particular species and age, needs excreta collecting trays
Solid walls	May give 'privacy', prevents draughts	May limit light and visibility, limits ventilation
No 'top'	Easy access to animal, may allow more light	Unless deep enough or close enough to next cage, may allow escape
'Top'	Often economises on space, allows easy provision of food and water	Limits accessibility, light and ventilation, needs to be a good fit and suitable for species to avoid escapes or injury
Doors and hatches	Must be easily worked by humans allowing sufficient access	
Catches	Must be easily worked by humans and not by the animal who has 24 hours a day to experiment (padlocks for primates) Must have as few working parts as possible and preferably no loose parts to get lost or parts operated by springs as these will rust	
'Squeeze' backs and perches	Special features of some primate cages	
Food hoppers and watering devices	Described in chapter 7, 'Feeding and Watering'	
Labelling	A tamper-proof system of labelling must be included	

heat away from the rabbit and its body temperature would drop. If the rabbit was housed at the same temperature, but in a wooden hutch, it would survive because the wood would act as an insulator enabling the rabbit to conserve its body heat.

In modern temperature controlled animal units the thermal conductivity of a material is a less important consideration.

- *Reactions with acids, alkalis and detergents at concentrations encountered in the animal units* – a number of chemicals are used in the animal unit (e.g. to descale and clean cages); the materials used to construct cages and pens must be able to resist their effects.
- *Ability to withstand repeated autoclaving.*

Most cages and pens are constructed from metal or plastic or a combination of both. Less common materials are wood and fibreglass. Properties of commonly used caging materials are summarised in Table 2.2.

ARRANGEMENT OF CAGES

A number of methods are used to arrange animal accommodation:

- *Racks* – can be mobile, free standing, fixed to the wall or suspended. Racks can be arranged along walls or in the centre of large rooms.
- *Shelves* – can be adjustable or in fixed position. They may also be cantilevered.
- *Batteries* – banks of cages connected to one another (e.g. chicken batteries).
- *Pens* – the room partitioned into areas.

Examples of cages, pens and racking are shown in Figs 2.1–2.9.

Table 2.2 Properties of caging materials.

Material	Properties	Examples of uses
Wood and wood products (including cardboard)	Construction of cages and boxes is easy with wood, however it is difficult to clean, impossible to sterilise and may rot. Wood is a good insulator but animals may gnaw it.	Limited use in the animal unit but can be used for travelling boxes, shelves, perches.
Metals • In general	Metals are strong, easily cleaned and will withstand autoclaving. They are good conductors of heat, which should not cause a problem in temperature controlled animal rooms. Most are heavy. They usually require specialist manufacturing techniques to construct. Animal or technician activity can generate noise.	
• Galvanised mild steel	This is mild steel that has been coated with a layer of zinc after manufacture. The zinc protects the underlying steel from rusting. Acids will remove the zinc coating exposing the underlying steel to rusting.	Although less popular than it was, this material is still used for racking, large cages and pens.
• Aluminium and its alloys	In contrast to other metals aluminium is relatively light in weight. It is a soft material, especially pure aluminium, and can be bent or even gnawed by some animals. Its surface may be pitted by alkaline agents.	Racking and rabbit cages.
• Stainless steel	Very strong material that is resistant to most substances found in animal units. It is very long lasting and the most expensive material used for caging.	Large cages for primates. Cage doors and tops, food hoppers and water bottle spouts.
• Brass	Material that is not often seen in modern animal houses, the brass has to be electroplated with chrome to prevent corrosion.	Water bottle tops and drinking valves.
Plastics • General	Light weight material that is a good insulator and resistant to damage by water and acids. It makes much less noise in use and if dropped than metal. The cost is low. They are made in one piece and are easy to stack. If there are sharp edges animals may be able to gnaw them. Traditional plastics become brittle with age and repeated autoclaving but modern high temperature/chemical tolerant plastics are much more resistant.	
• Polycarbonate	A clear plastic that will withstand autoclaving at 121°C. It becomes discoloured and brittle with repeated treatments. Detergents make this material cloudy.	Commonly used for rodent boxes.
• Polypropylene	Translucent plastic that can be autoclaved at 121°C. It discolours with age.	Rat and mouse boxes.
• Polyethylene (polythene, alkathene)	This plastic is deformed by high temperatures.	Rabbit cages.
• Polysulfone	Transparent, slightly smoke coloured material. Withstands autoclaving at temperatures up to 130°C. Heat and chemical resistant.	Caging.
• Polystyrene	Cheap and disposable. It is brittle and cannot be autoclaved.	Disposable cages.
• Melamine, Bakelite	Hard but brittle plastic.	Water bottle spouts.
Glass resin polymer (fibreglass)	GRP can be used to make small quantities of special cages. The material is a good insulator and strong but it may fracture if dropped. It can be easily repaired.	Beds and transport boxes for dogs and cats.
Glass	Transparent and impervious to all chemicals used in the animal house. It is fragile and is easily broken, resulting in dangerous sharp edges.	Drinking bottles and metabolism cages.

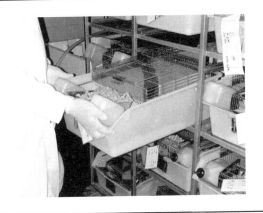

Fig. 2.1 Polypropylene rat cage.

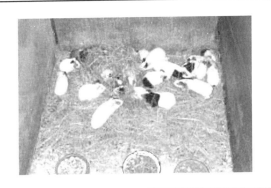

Fig. 2.4 Guinea pig floor pen.

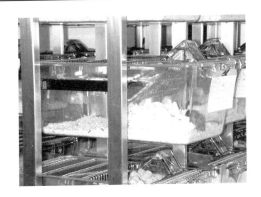

Fig. 2.2 Polycarbonate mouse cage.

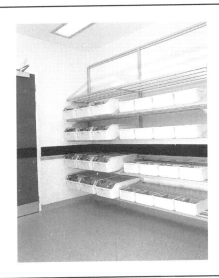

Fig. 2.5 Rodent cages arranged on shelves.

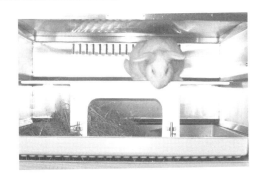

Fig. 2.3 Rabbit cage – stainless steel sides and furniture with plastic tray.

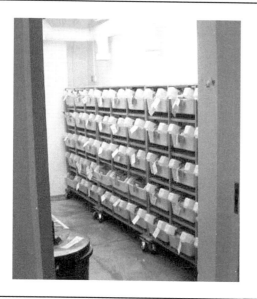

Fig. 2.6 Rodent cages arranged on a rack.

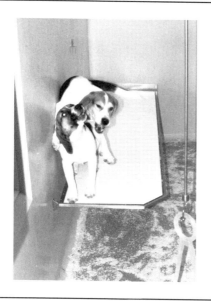

Fig. 2.7 Dog pen with shelf.

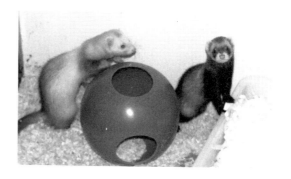

Fig. 2.8 Ferret pen.

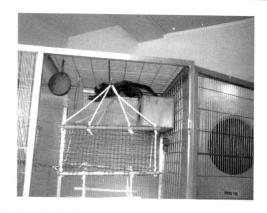

Fig. 2.9 Marmoset cage.

The factors which limit the number of animals which may be housed within one room include:

1. The type of cages, pens, racking and shelves available.
2. The space needed to service the cages and to work with the animals.
3. The density at which the animals will enjoy good health (which will be affected by ventilation and methods of husbandry).

Chapter 3
The Animal House

An animal house is any structure that accommodates animals and the service equipment and facilities necessary to maintain them. In the UK facilities intended to house animals used or bred for scientific procedures must hold a Certificate of Designation (see Chapter 13) issued by the Home Office. This certificate will only be given if the facilities reach the high standard described in the current edition of the Home Office Code of Practice for the Housing and Care of Animals Used in Scientific Procedures (CoPSP) or the Code of Practice for Breeding and Supplying Establishments (CoPB).

Designated animal units range in size from one or two rodent rooms to facilities accommodating thousands of animals of many different species. Whatever the size of the unit the aim must be to provide a stable environment so that the animals' physiological and behavioural needs are met and they are able to be bred and studied for experimental purposes (Figs 3.1, 3.2).

Ideally animal houses should be purpose built and should be physically separate from other buildings. This minimises the risk of animals being disturbed by extraneous noise and it increases security. The design of the unit should provide maximum flexibility so that changing from one species to another can be done without major alterations. The rooms should contain the minimum amount of fixed equipment, all surfaces should be covered with an impervious material and all junctions should be coved so that places where dust can collect are minimised and the room can be easily cleaned. A facility is usually divided into areas so that activities can be separated (cleaning, breeding, experimental) and into individual rooms so that species and studies can be kept separately. Breeding animals must be disturbed as little as possible so they are usually isolated from experimental animals and other parts of the unit.

Animals that are brought into the unit may have to undergo a period of quarantine to ensure they are free from disease-causing organisms before they are allowed contact with established animals. The quarantine unit must be isolated from other rooms.

Areas set aside for cage cleaning, air conditioning plant and other potentially noisy activities should be situated as far away from the animals as possible to minimise disturbance.

Basic services must be provided in animal units. These include heat, ventilation, light, power, water and drainage. Drains must be large enough to deal with the volume of effluent produced in an animal unit. Drains should be fitted with a mesh filter (catch pot) to catch sawdust. The filter needs to be emptied at regular intervals. U-bends, which prevent the escape of sewer gases, must not be allowed to dry out.

Power in animal units is provided by electricity. The other services listed above are dealt with later in the book.

BARRIERS

Animals within a unit must be protected from infectious organisms. Micro-organisms can enter an animal unit in a number of ways including:

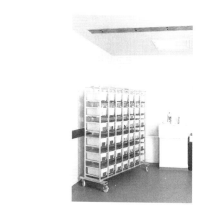

Fig. 3.1 Typical animal room with wheeled rack and sink.

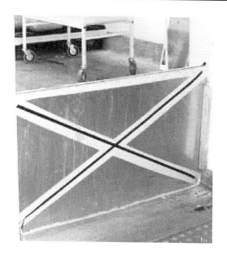

Fig. 3.3 Rodent barrier which prevents rodents entering or leaving the room.

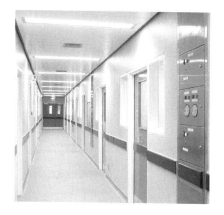

Fig. 3.2 Animal unit corridor showing environmental monitoring panel.

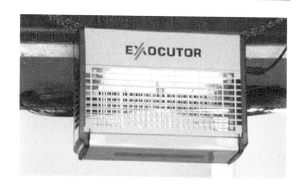

Fig. 3.4 Ultra violet insect electrocuter.

- On imported animals.
- In food and bedding.
- On staff.
- On air.

When animals are kept in large numbers, in a confined area, infectious diseases spread very rapidly. In order to prevent them entering and travelling around the unit barriers are erected. A barrier is any physical arrangement, procedures or routine set up with the intent of minimising the likelihood of contamination of the animal with unwanted micro-organisms. Examples of barriers are:

- Physical separation from other buildings.
- Restricted entry of personnel.
- Use of protective clothing.
- Showering into the unit.
- Rodent and insect barriers (Figs 3.3, 3.4).
- Routine use of disinfectants.

- Appropriate use of sterilisation procedures.
- Air conditioning with filtered air and pressure differentials.

All animal units institute barriers but the extent of them depends on the nature of the work that goes on in the unit and the length of time the animals are kept. Where animals are housed for a short time the risk of them contracting and suffering disease is low. In this situation it may be only necessary to restrict entry to non essential personnel, require staff to wear protective clothing, institute routine cage cleaning and disinfection programmes and have filtered air conditioning.

If the work within the unit involves long term studies it is essential, from both an animal welfare and from a scientific point of view, that disease organisms are kept out. In this case more stringent barriers must be instituted. In addition to the measures mentioned above anyone entering the unit may be required to shower and dress in sterilised clothing before entering. All goods would be sterilised on entry. Air supply would be filtered and at positive pressure to the outside to prevent airborne micro-organisms entering. All entry points would be protected with insecticutors and rodent traps. These types of animal houses are called full barrier units.

Whatever the type of animal unit the objectives remain the same – to provide a protective environment that can be reliably maintained and yet permit man controlled access to the animal.

Chapter 4
Environment

All that surrounds or exerts an effect on the animal forms its environment. The conditions immediately surrounding the animal, e.g. the cage, pen or the nest, are referred to as the micro-environment. The term macro-environment is used when referring to the conditions outside the micro-environment.

Unlike wild animals, those kept in laboratory animal units have a more limited opportunity to control their own environment; they are dependent on man to control it for them. Many species or strains of animals used in scientific procedures have been so altered by selective breeding (e.g. the nude mouse) that they would be unlikely to survive outside the controlled environment of the animal unit.

Animals differ in the way they respond to their environment and there are major differences in the way animals and man respond to the same environment. Conditions that man might find tolerable may not be acceptable to animals. For example in most laboratory mammals smell is a much more important sense than it is in man and they are able to hear sounds at a much higher pitch than man. These and other differences must be accounted for when establishing a suitable environment for them.

The environment of laboratory animals includes:

- The cage, bedding, diet, water, other animals.
- Temperature, relative humidity, day length, light intensity.
- Air (the oxygen, carbon dioxide, water vapour, ammonia and dust content).

- Routine care procedures, noise.
- Man.
- Breeding systems or experimental procedures.
- Micro-organisms, diseases and treatments.

Some of these factors are easy to control, others much less so. The factors listed above that are not discussed in detail in this chapter are covered elsewhere.

MAN

Man controls all aspects of the living conditions of animals and as such is totally responsible for their environment; animals suffer if staff are uncaring and unobservant. More directly when animals are handled for routine maintenance tasks, e.g. when changing cages or for the assessment of health status, good handling techniques minimise the amount of disturbance. Poor technique may create resentful or aggressive animals and can lead to injury.

OTHER ANIMALS

Most species react adversely to being caged singly; they appear to miss social contact, e.g. being able to groom one another. They may become aggressive and develop abnormal behavioural patterns. When animals are housed in groups, whether for breeding or experimental purposes, the groupings are unnatural as man, not the animals, chooses their cage mates. Initially in new groups there may be some fighting but a hierarchy is rapidly established and the animals soon settle down. However new groups must be watched carefully as bullying may occur. Once a group has been established new animals should not be added as the established animals may attack the newcomer.

Some strains of animals are very aggressive and special care must be taken when these are group housed.

Group housing will increase the amounts of waste, the temperature and the relative humidity within the cage. Higher levels of ammonia will be produced creating an unpleasant environment and increasing the risk of disease.

Acceptable stocking densities are given in the Codes of Practice.

LIGHT

Most laboratory animal accommodation is built without windows. All light is artificial and therefore can be strictly controlled. The light environment is made up of three elements – intensity, photoperiod and wavelength – all of which can affect the well-being of laboratory animals, breeding performance and experimental results.

Intensity

Light intensity is measured in units of lux. Natural light in full sun can produce a reading of about 100 000 lux falling to 20 lux in full moonlight. The Home Office CoP states that levels of 350–400 lux measured at bench height are suitable for routine experimental and laboratory activities. However intensity within the room will vary; near the light source it may be as high as 700 lux and in a cage at the bottom of a rodent rack could be as low as 10 lux. There is little evidence on the intensity that animals prefer although experimental evidence suggests that rats produce more litters when kept at 100 lux.

Many laboratory species are nocturnal or crepuscular animals so their eyes are adapted to function in dim light. Exposure to bright light can cause retinal damage. The situation is made worse if the animals are albinos as they have no protective pigment in their eyes. Damage of this kind has been seen to occur in rodents housed at the top of a

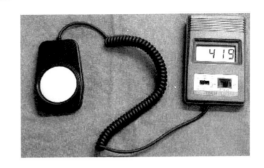

Fig. 4.1 Light meter.

rack. Light intensity is measured with a light meter (Fig. 4.1).

Animals benefit from situations where a two level light system operates, the higher intensity being used to provide staff with adequate light to carry out their duties and a lower level to simulate dawn and dusk.

Photoperiod

Photoperiod is the length of time the animals are exposed to light during the day. The reproductive cycles of many species are controlled by day length as the stimulus of light affects circulating hormone levels. In natural light some species will stop or slow their reproductive cycles at certain times of the year as the length of the light period changes (e.g. hamster). These seasonal variations often disappear with a constant photoperiod of adequate length, e.g. 12 hours light and 12 hours dark. Manipulating light periods can stimulate seasonal breeders like the ferret to become reproductively active outside their normal season. In some circumstances it may be possible to change the lighting regime so that animal activities that normally occur at night are performed during the working day. For instance, Syrian hamsters are most sexually active approximately one hour after night fall. Adjusting the photoperiod so that the lights go off at mid-day may be convenient when hand mating systems have to be used.

Continuous darkness has the effect of lengthening the oestrous cycle in many animals and continuous light can produce continuous oestrus. Both situations will result in a drop in breeding productivity and eventual cessation of breeding.

Wavelength

The wavelength of light determines colour perception. There is no evidence that any laboratory species, other than cats, some birds and primates can distinguish colour. However, there is some experimental evidence to show that ultra violet light has a beneficial effect on animals housed indoors.

Vision

There are species differences in visual perception. Some species are unable to judge distance, e.g. sheep can be frightened by a movement a long way off. The hamster is more sensitive to movement than detail and so appears short-sighted.

NOISE

Noise is unwanted sound. Levels of noise should be kept low so that animals are not startled and so they can communicate by sound without interference. Sound has two properties, intensity and frequency.

Intensity and frequency

Sound intensity (or volume) is measured on a logarithmic scale in deciBels (dB). The pitch of a sound depends on its frequency. The higher the frequency the higher the pitch. Frequency is measured in hertz (Hz).

Not all species are sensitive to the same sound frequencies. Humans with good hearing can hear a range of frequencies from 0.2–20 kHz, but are most sensitive to sounds in the range of 0.5–5 kHz. These frequencies appear to be louder than other frequencies to the human ear, even though the intensity is the same. Humans cannot perceive sounds lower than 0.2 kHz (infrasound) and higher than 20 kHz (ultrasound) at all.

For this reason straight dB measurement is not very useful when assessing how annoying a sound is to humans as it treats all sound the same whatever its frequency. To overcome this problem sound meters have been developed that filter sound so that extra consideration is given to the frequencies that humans are most sensitive to. Measurements on this scale are called dB (A weighted scale) or dBA.

Rats are sensitive to sound in a frequency range which extends from 0.25–76 kHz and they are most sensitive between 35 and 40 kHz. Cats are able to perceive sound in a range from 0.0075–91 kHz with peak sensitivity of 1–40 kHz.

Even though animals have different frequency sensitivity to humans the Home Office Codes of Practice quote noise levels in dBA and state that an unoccupied animal room should have noise levels below 50 dBA.

Long lasting noise at high intensity, or of a frequency which annoys the species, or sudden irregular noises produce stress that may be exhibited by changes in behaviour and/or breeding performance. In some susceptible strains noise can cause fits (audiogenic seizure).

The disturbing effects of noise may be limited in a number of ways:

- *The design of the animal house* – of particular importance where species which make a lot of noise themselves (e.g. dogs and monkeys) are housed. The building must either absorb the noise or noisy animals must be housed away from quieter species.
- *Appropriate apparatus* – soft shoes for staff, cushioned floors, plastic bins, rubber-wheeled trolleys, 'Silentone' fire alarms.
- *Arrangement of routines* – locating noisy jobs away from animals. Carrying out jobs that produce ultrasound (filling water bottles, using vacuum cleaners or VDU screens) away from animals.

Sounds produced by animals, which are associated with courtship, mothering, excitement, aggression and defence are a necessary part of their communication which can be frustrated by high ambient noise levels. Low level 'piped' music is used in some animal houses either to mask other noises or for its claimed soothing effects.

Sound with intensities of 90 dBA or more for a period of time will cause permanent hearing loss in humans. These levels could be generated in a kennel at feeding time. Ear protectors should be worn in these circumstances.

TEMPERATURE

Ectotherms, i.e. reptiles, amphibia, fish and invertebrates, have a metabolic rate which is more or less dependent on ambient temperature. Most laboratory species, i.e. mammals and birds, are endothermic which means that they regulate their body temperatures within a narrow range by varying their metabolic rate.

Mammals are kept at a temperature that allows them to lose heat to their surroundings when they produce more heat than is needed to maintain their body temperature. Heat losses are incurred by the animals through conduction, convection and radiation, and evaporation of water from the airways and skin causes cooling by a process called latent heat of vaporisation (see Figs 4.2–4.5):

- Conduction – heat lost through the cage bottom (limited by choice of materials).
- Convection – heat lost to the atmosphere (limited by the coat and the elimination of draughts).
- Radiation – heat lost in the form of infra red radiation to the surroundings (uncontrollable).
- Latent heat of vaporisation of water – breathing/panting, sweating (in a few species) or becoming wet will cause an animal to lose heat. Water needs energy to evaporate from the surface of the animal. It gets this energy from the animal body so as the moisture evaporates the animal loses heat energy and gets colder. Heat loss by this method is limited by high relative humidity, the coat and the elimination of draughts.

Heat losses are controlled by physical, physiological and behavioural means. Conservation of heat is achieved by constricting surface blood capillaries, seasonal thickening of the coat, piloerec-

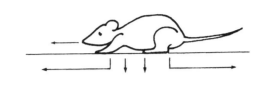

Fig. 4.2 Conduction.

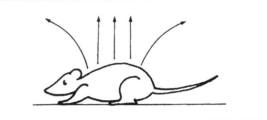

Fig. 4.3 Convection.

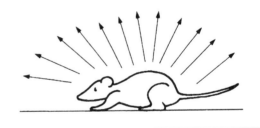

Fig. 4.4 Radiation.

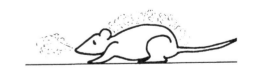

Fig. 4.5 Latent heat of vaporisation of water.

tion (fluffing of the coat), posture (sitting hunched up) or nest building. The rate of heat loss may be increased by dilating surface blood capillaries, sweating (most laboratory animals are only capable of sweating from the paws), panting, hyperventilation and posture (lying spread out).

In the wild, mammals can compensate to some extent for sub-optimal temperatures but this entails a greater expenditure of energy. The development of better insulation such as thicker or longer coats and more substantial layers of fat may occur prior to winter. Extremes of temperature would ultimately adversely affect the health of most animals and would certainly affect the development or even the survival of the unweaned. In the laboratory an increase in dietary intake may be observed in mammals kept at just a few degrees below the optimum to compensate for heat loss.

Smaller animals have a large surface area in proportion to their body mass and are therefore more prone to losing too much heat. Generally, the larger the animal, the lower its optimum environmental temperature.

The Home Office Code of Practice states that temperatures within animal rooms should be carefully controlled and monitored at least once a day. The optimum temperatures stated are:

- Laboratory rodents   19° to 23°C
- Rabbits   16° to 20°C
- Guinea pigs   16° to 23°C
- Dogs, cats, ferrets   15° to 24°C

The temperature should not fluctuate more than 4°C, with the whole of the band within the temperature range. At these room air temperatures, temperature-related stress to the animal and effects on experimental results should be minimised.

HUMIDITY

Humidity refers to the amount of water vapour in the air. Relative humidity (RH) is the amount of water vapour contained in a volume of air expressed as a percentage of the amount of water vapour that would be present in the same volume of air saturated with water vapour, at the same temperature.

As with all environmental factors wide variations in humidity or long periods at either low or high levels will stress animals and may create the conditions in which diseases can develop, e.g. low humidity may cause a condition known as ringtail in young rats and encourages some types of respiratory infections. The CoPSP states that the relative humidity in animal rooms should normally be maintained at 55% +/– 10% and that prolonged periods below 40% and above 70% should be avoided.

Temperature and humidity are closely linked. Warm air can hold more moisture than dry air so that if the temperature rises the relative humidity will fall even though the amount of water in the atmosphere remains constant.

AIR

Animals must be provided with sufficient amounts of clean fresh air. Waste gases, excess heat, moisture and other unwanted substances produced by the animals and animal room activities must be removed from animal rooms. Failure to do so will adversely affect the animals.

Ventilation system

Control of temperature, humidity and air quality is a function of the ventilation system. Most animal units will have a ventilation system capable of:

- Regulating temperature and humidity within prescribed limits.
- Reducing the levels and spread of odours, noxious gases, dust and infectious agents.
- Providing sufficient air of an appropriate quality.

Air is supplied to the room through ducts so that each animal is supplied with fresh air but no animal is in a draught. The rate at which fresh air is supplied to the room will depend on the stocking density of the room but a fully stocked rodent room will normally require 15–20 air changes per hour. Most rooms containing animals free from infectious organisms are supplied with air at a faster rate than it is removed from the room so that the room is at positive pressure to the outside. This ensures that airborne organisms are not able to get into the room. Rooms where infected animals are housed are kept at negative pressure to the outside so that airborne organisms cannot escape from the room.

In addition to ventilating whole rooms, independent ventilated racks are available where each cage is fitted with its own filtered air supply. The cages have a filtered top and are able to be kept at positive or negative pressure. The cages are removed to a cleaning station for cleaning (Fig. 4.6).

MONITORING THE ENVIRONMENT

It is necessary to monitor the physical environment within the animal unit to ensure the system is working properly and delivering the levels required. Animals will suffer in an adverse environment and experimental results also vary in unstable conditions. For these reasons the Animals (Scientific Procedures) Act 1986 places a duty on Named Animal Care and Welfare Officers to keep records of environmental values.

Most laboratory animal facilities are fitted with building management systems (BMS) (Fig. 4.7). These comprise electronic sensors, arranged in the rooms, which collect information on temperature, humidity etc. and feed it to a computer. The com-

puter not only keeps a continuous record of these values but also gives warnings if any value falls outside a pre-set limit.

Even though computerised monitoring systems are available manual methods still have an important role to play in ensuring a stable environment. Monitoring must still go on if the computerised

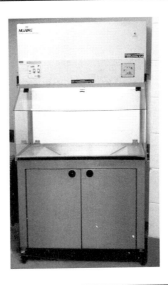

Fig. 4.6 Cage cleaning station.

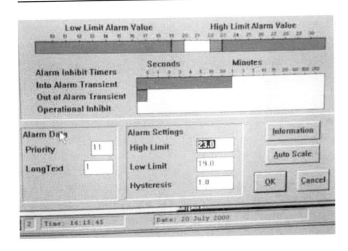

Fig. 4.7 Computer screen of building management system showing temperature setting.

system fails. Manual methods can also be used to check the accuracy of the electronic system.

Manual method of measuring temperature

Temperature is usually measured in degrees Celsius (°C). Many methods are available for measuring and monitoring the air temperatures, e.g. liquid in glass thermometers; thermocouples; bi-metallic strip thermometers and thermographs.

Temperature should be monitored at least once each day and should be checked at the same time each day. The maximum and minimum temperatures reached within each monitoring period should be noted so that the extremes of temperature variation are known. A simple instrument in common use is the maximum-minimum thermometer that shows the highest and lowest temperature reached since resetting and the room temperature at the time of reading (Figs 4.8, 4.9).

Siting maximum-minimum thermometers

Ideally, the maximum-minimum thermometer should be placed in a position that is most likely to show the conditions experienced by the animals, i.e. away from sources of heat (heating systems, the sink and the animals themselves) and away from the cooling effect of local draughts (doors), at the average height of the animals in the room (halfway up a rack of cages or near the floor if the animals are housed in pens).

Manual method of measuring relative humidity

Relative humidity can be measured using the wet and dry bulb hygrometer, adsorption hygrometer, hair hygrometer and hygrographs.

Stationary or rotating (whirling) wet and dry bulb hygrometers are often used in animal units. Both instruments consist of two identical mercury in glass thermometers set side by side in the same plane against graduated scales. The bulb of one of the thermometers is connected to a wick, which is immersed in a reservoir of distilled water that has to be topped up periodically (Fig. 4.10). Only dis-

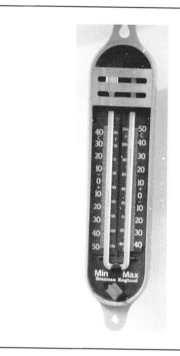

Fig. 4.8 Maximum and minimum thermometer.

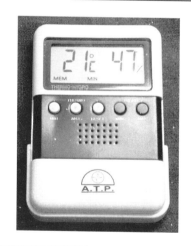

Fig. 4.9 Electronic maximum and minimum thermometer and hygrometer.

tilled or demineralised water should be used in this reservoir as the mineral salts that are present in tap water will eventually clog the wick and restrict the flow of water to the wet bulb. In the whirling version the thermometers and reservoir are enclosed in a frame which can be rapidly rotated around a handle. The whirling hygrometer (Fig. 4.11) should be rotated with an even velocity for about 30 seconds. It should be read (wet bulb first) and the procedure repeated until two wet bulb readings are the same.

These instruments rely on the evaporation of moisture from the wet bulb to the atmosphere. In order to evaporate the water needs energy and it obtains this from the thermometer, so the evaporation produces a lower temperature than that recorded on the dry bulb. The dryer the atmosphere the more water will evaporate and so the lower the temperature reading from the wet bulb will be. The relative humidity can then be read from a hygrometric table (Table 4.1) or graph.

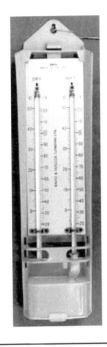

Fig. 4.10 Masons hygrometer.

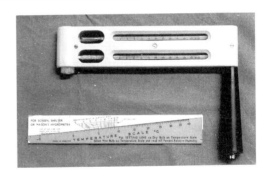

Fig. 4.11 Whirling hygrometer.

Example: Wet bulb 15.5°C.
             Dry bulb 21.0°C.

The wet bulb depression is calculated by subtracting the wet bulb temperature from the dry bulb temperature in Table 4.1, in this case 5.5°C. This figure is located on the x axis (the horizontal line) on the chart. The dry bulb temperature is located on the y axis (the vertical line) on the chart. Where the two lines bisect the relative humidity level is recorded, in this case 53% RH.

Hair hygrometers work on the principle that hair expands and contracts in response to the amount of water in the atmosphere. One end of the hair is kept fixed and the other is attached to a lever. When the atmosphere is dry the hair contracts and the lever is moved one way. In damp atmospheres the hair expands and the lever is moved in the opposite direction.

Although maximum-minimum thermometers and whirling hygrometers are useful, they do not record the time of day and the duration of any fluctuations. These can be recorded by using a thermohygrograph (Fig. 4.12).

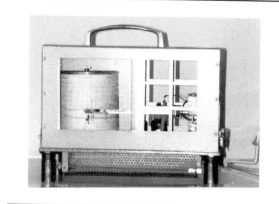

Fig. 4.12 Thermohygrograph – consists of a bimetalic strip to record temperature and hair to record humidity, both being recorded on a rotating drum.

Table 4.1 Hygrometric table.

Depression of wet bulb in degrees Celsius

T	2.5	3.0	3.5	4.0	4.5	5.0	5.5	6.0	6.5	7.0	7.5	8.0	8.5
24	79	75	71	68	64	60	57	53	50	46	43	39	36
23	79	75	71	67	63	59	56	52	48	45	41	38	35
22	78	74	70	66	62	58	54	51	47	43	40	36	33
21	78	73	69	65	61	57	53	49	45	42	38	35	31
20	77	73	68	64	60	56	52	48	44	40	36	33	29
19	76	72	67	63	59	55	50	46	42	38	34	31	27
18	76	71	66	62	58	53	49	45	41	36	32	29	25
17	75	70	65	61	56	52	47	43	39	34	30	26	22
16	74	69	64	60	55	50	46	41	37	32	28	24	20
15	73	68	63	58	53	49	44	39	35	30	26	21	17

Dry bulb temp. °C

Chapter 5
Routine Animal House Procedures

A routine is an established method of completing a task or series of tasks. Routines are prepared for all the work necessary to maintain laboratory animals because:

- They ensure no task gets forgotten.
- They enable work to be planned efficiently.
- Animals become accustomed to the work and are less disturbed by it.

Basic routines are the same for all animals and all types of unit; they include:

- Checking the environment (temperature, humidity, air pressure, peculiar smells).
- Checking the condition of the animals.
- Feeding and watering.
- Cleaning out pens, cages or trays.
- Changing and cleaning cages.
- Cleaning equipment.
- Cleaning the room and its fittings.

The basic elements of the routine are similar but they must be adapted to fit the needs of each species, method of housing and type of work. Differences that affect the routines include:

- The amount and consistency of faeces (dogs wet and smelly need cleaning at least once a day, mice relatively dry need cleaning only twice a week).
- Type of food (dry pellets can stay in hopper for several days, wet food or fresh food must be changed every day).
- Cage stocking density (multi-occupied cages

need cleaning more often than singly housed animals).
- Type of work (breeding units need pairing, weaning etc. included into the routine).
- Experimental demands.

BEDDING MATERIAL

One of the most important routine tasks is to ensure the animals are kept clean and comfortable. This involves regular cleaning and changing of bedding material (the word 'litter' is often used to mean the same thing as bedding). Bedding material may be placed on the floor of a solid bottomed cage or pen and so be in direct contact with the animal, or it may be used to line a tray underneath a cage and so be separated from the animal by a grid or perforated floor. The appropriate bedding must be selected for each situation.

The ideal bedding material

The properties expected of an ideal bedding material are:

- *Harmless to animals* – i.e. non-toxic (containing no poisonous material), non-injurious (containing no sharp pieces to wound), dust-free, free from living organisms (especially those that cause disease – this implies it must be sterilisable).
- *Absorbent* – to soak up urine and spilled water so animals keep dry and to cover faeces to prevent animals becoming soiled.
- *A thermal insulator* – to reduce conduction of

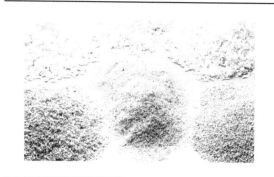

Fig. 5.1 Bedding materials.

body heat through the floor of the cage (insulating properties decrease with wetness).

- *Comfortable.*
- *Readily available* – so that sufficient quantities of the required quality can be obtained throughout the year.
- *Packed conveniently* for handling and storage.
- *Easily disposable* – preferably by incineration as large volumes are involved and some may be chemically or biologically contaminated.
- *Reasonably priced* – true cost is a function of the purchase price, storage costs, amount used, how frequently it has to be replaced and cost of disposal.

In addition to the above, bedding materials should be inedible, should not stain and should be easy to remove and handle when cleaning out (Fig. 5.1).

Materials

Wood products – sawdust, wood chips, shavings

Wood for bedding should only come from soft, white wood (conifers), because some hardwoods contain toxic chemicals such as phenols that could be absorbed by the animals. It is advisable to purchase wood products from specialist suppliers who ensure the wood has not been chemically treated with preservatives and have analyses carried out to determine heavy metal content and microbiological status. Specialist manufacturers

will also grade products to the desired particle size, and exclude dust and large, potentially harmful pieces.

Wood materials are dried to reduce the moisture content to less than 10%, so they will absorb a considerable amount of moisture before they become soggy. The degree of absorbency is related to the particle size, shavings being less absorbent than smaller sized particles. Wood itself is a poor conductor of heat, but in particle form the air trapped between the particles makes it a very good insulator.

A continuous supply of wood products is available of the quality and in the packaging (e.g. compressed, shrink-wrapped or steam permeable bags) the user requires. Soiled bedding is easy to dispose of by incineration.

Wood products can be used as contact or non-contact bedding. The cost of the material depends on the quality of the product and the extent of the quality control analysis that is required.

Peat moss

Peat moss is a naturally occurring material produced by the bacterial decay of vegetable matter in stagnant deoxygenated water. This process results in a chemically inert substance that has a low pH which inhibits bacterial growth. It may contain sharp objects and it will make animals dirty, so it can only be used as non-contact bedding.

Dry peat is capable of holding more water than sawdust, though completely dry peat may be difficult to obtain. When dry it is a good thermal insulator and is readily burnt in an incinerator.

Although peat is dug and dried on a seasonal basis, supplies can be obtained throughout the year. The low pH slows the bacterial breakdown of urine and faeces and therefore delays the release of ammonia. This, in addition to its absorbency, means that animals kept on peat do not require cleaning out as often as those kept on sawdust, so a given amount of peat will last longer than an equivalent amount of sawdust and it can be cost effective to use despite its higher purchase price.

Two factors preclude its use:

- It always looks dirty and contaminates animals and staff.
- It is a finite resource. There is much concern about the destruction of irreplaceable peat bogs to satisfy the horticultural trade. Where there are other materials that can be used there is no reason to use peat.

Paper products

Sheets of absorbent paper are available cut to fit cage trays (Fig. 5.2). The manufacturing process ensures the paper has a very low microbial load, it is easily stored, can be sterilised if necessary, and can be disposed of by incineration. It can only be used as a non-contact bedding as animals will tear it up.

A major advantage of using paper is the very low levels of dust and the consequent reduction of allergens. Further advantages are that it is easier to clean out, estimate food wastage and investigate urine and faeces.

Other specifically manufactured paper bedding materials are available. These materials are cut and folded to provide a soft, comfortable substrate with good insulating properties. They can be used as contact bedding for dogs and other larger animals. Urine runs through the material to the base of the cage and is absorbed from the bottom up, keeping the top layer dry. Paper is readily in-

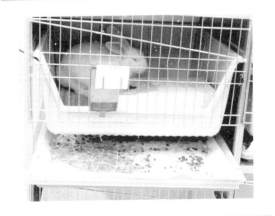

Fig. 5.2 Paper sheet in rabbit cage tray.

cinerated. Because the material is specifically manufactured its quality is constant and can be assured.

Corn cob

Corn cob is produced by crushing a maize cob after the maize has been extracted and grading into required sizes. The bedding is a good insulator and appears to be comfortable for the animals. Urine drains through the bedding to the bottom of the cage and is absorbed by the bottom layer of corn cob, keeping the animals clean and dry. The absorbency of corn cob is so good that animals need cleaning out less often than those on wood products. It has low dust levels.

NESTING MATERIALS

The qualities of an ideal nesting material are similar to those of an ideal bedding material but with the following differences:

- The animal should be able to construct an adequate nest from it.
- It should not absorb moisture but should allow it to run through to the bedding material so the animal stays dry.
- It should provide privacy.

Materials

Straw

Even the softest straw is likely to be too harsh for small laboratory species.

Hay

Hay is a natural nesting material and food for many species. In the animal unit care must be taken because it may contain coarse plants such as thistles and could be contaminated with mould, bacteria, chemicals or other wildlife.

Good quality meadow hay should be free from weeds and will provide a soft nesting material for animals; however all hay contains microbiological contaminants and should be sterilised by autoclaving or irradiation before being given

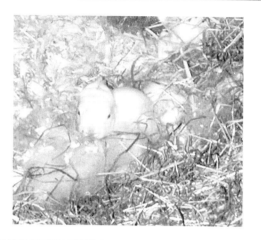

Fig. 5.3 Young rabbits in hay and rabbit fur nest.

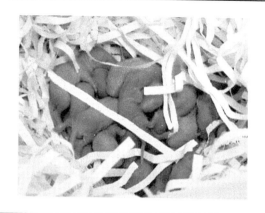

Fig. 5.4 Mouse pups in shredded paper nest.

to laboratory animals. Rabbits will build nests with hay (Fig. 5.3) and it gives privacy to guinea pigs. Both species will eat it so it will need frequent replenishment.

Wood-wool

Soft grade wood-wool makes a good nest for mice, rats, hamsters and carnivores. If the material is too harsh it could damage new born animals. Wood-wool is less absorbent than other wood products but otherwise has the same properties.

Paper products

Many types of paper are used as nesting materials including absorbent cellulose wadding, tissue paper towels, newsprint (newspaper before it has been printed) and tea-bag paper. Paper can be given already shredded (Fig. 5.4) or as a sheet that the animals shred for themselves. Nesting materials need to be replaced regularly or they become soiled and wet.

Cotton fibre

Sheets of cotton fibre divided into 5 × 5 cm pieces can be added to the cage so the animal can shred

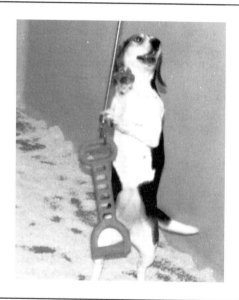

Fig. 5.5 Dog exercising with rubber toy.

and construct nests from them. The material is soft, non-irritating, inert and non-digestible.

ENVIRONMENTAL ENRICHMENT

Nesting materials provide an easy way to enrich an animal's environment. Building the nest provides occupation and exercise, the finished nest

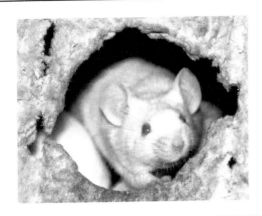

Fig. 5.6 Mouse 'Des. Res'.

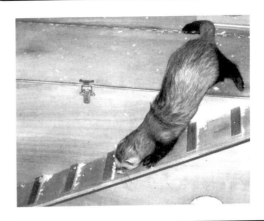

Fig. 5.8 Ferret using climbing box.

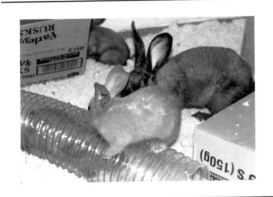

Fig. 5.7 Rabbits in floor pens with enriched environment.

provides privacy and a choice of environments (either the nest or the rest of the cage). Other materials can be easily added to a cage to increase the activity and interest for animals without impeding experimental results. Examples are rodent chew sticks, compressed grass sticks for rabbits and guinea pigs, and rodent or rabbit tunnels. Balls, imitation bones, rings and other similar materials can be provided for carnivores and primates. These are non-toxic, have no nutrient value and can be sterilised.

Animals benefit from any item of interest in their environment but the cage or pen should never be so filled that movement of the animal is restricted (Figs 5.5, 5.6, 5.7, 5.8).

Chapter 6
Hygiene

Hygiene is concerned with the maintenance of health. Hygienic conditions are achieved by the use of routine cleaning, sterilisation and disinfection. The aim of these routines is to reduce the levels of substances likely to cause allergic reactions (see Chapter 15) and the numbers of organisms that could cause disease, thereby providing a healthy environment for animals and people within the animal facility.

The organisms that cause disease are viruses, bacteria, fungi (moulds and yeasts) and invertebrate parasites, their eggs and larvae (protozoa, worms, insects and arachnids). Of these, bacterial spores are the most difficult to destroy. Spores are formed by some groups of bacteria when their environment becomes hostile; they are very resilient and can exist in spore form for very long periods. When spores find a suitable environment they begin to grow and reproduce again.

CLEANING

To achieve hygienic conditions appropriate cleaning regimes must be applied in an appropriate way. Inadequate attention to detail or the use of unsuitable cleaning agents or disinfectants will result in the spread of agents believed to be removed or destroyed.

Cleaning regimes in animal rooms have three major objectives:

- To remove, destroy or contain contaminated objects.
- To provide clean conditions for the animals.
- To provide conditions acceptable to workers.

All cleaning processes involve moving dirt from one place to another. Efficient methods are those which remove the dirt from the environment of the animals to the outside, e.g. via a drain or in a polythene bag to the incinerator.

A combination of methods are employed to clean the unit. Factors involved in the choice of methods are:

- The desired state of cleanliness, e.g. sterile, disinfected or merely free from obvious dirt.
- Properties of the surface being cleaned, e.g. absorbency, resistance to scratching.
- Nature of the item and the safety of the animals and the operators, e.g. electrical equipment such as light and power fittings, electronic balances and electric clippers.
- Nature of dirt to be removed, e.g. grease, dust and limescale.
- Availability of services, e.g. water, drains, power, vacuum and specialised equipment.
- Properties of any chemicals used, e.g. toxicity, staining, corrosiveness and rinsing ability.
- Experimental or special requirements, e.g. the use of a chemical recommended by the Ministry of Agriculture, Fisheries and Food in quarantine facilities.

Each animal unit devises procedures for cleaning which take account of all of these factors in order to achieve the desired state of cleanliness of surfaces and items of equipment.

Cleaning agents

A cleaning agent is any physical or chemical means that removes dirt from an article or surface. Water is commonly used to remove surface dirt. Its efficiency is affected by:

- The temperature it is used at, being more effective at high temperatures.
- Its physical form – liquid, spray or steam.
- The contact time – soaking in water often releases stubborn dirt.
- Its method of application – immersion, hosing or high pressure hosing.
- The addition of agitation or scrubbing.

Chemical cleaning agents can be added to water to enhance its efficiency, for instance soaps and detergents break up fatty materials so that water can wash them away.

Cleaning methods

Methods employed within animal units for achieving cleanliness, with some of their principal advantages and disadvantages, are listed in Table 6.1.

Cleaning cages and pens

How often cages are changed and bedding is cleaned out or replenished is determined by many interrelated factors which include:

- Cage (site, size and design).
- Animals (numbers, species, site and behaviour of individuals).
- Type of diet and the methods of presentation of food and water.
- Amount and type of bedding used.
- Likelihood of the presence of pests and parasites.
- Environmental conditions (temperature and ventilation).
- Experimental requirements.
- Cost of materials and labour.
- Interference caused to the animal's environment and behaviour.

The cleaning interval selected is a compromise between the factors above. For instance, it is important to provide a clean environment for animals and to ensure they are not exposed to high levels of ammonia in the cage. However, changing cages too frequently disturbs the animals and they take

Table 6.1 Methods of cleaning.

Method	Principal advantages	Principal disadvantages
Dusting	Quick, looks good	Transfers dirt from one place to another
Sweeping	Quick, looks good	Creates dust
Vacuuming	Removes dirt from the environment	Noisy unless the motor is outside the animal room
Wet mopping	Contains dust by wetting	Leaves smears of dirt, raises RH and creates slippery floors
Hosing	Removes dirt to the drain	Raises RH, takes a long time to dry, requires drains
High pressure hosing[1]	Removes stubborn dirt	As above plus greater splashback and aerosols, may spread dirt. Can injure user
High pressure hosing with steam	As above, heat energy kills some organisms *in situ*	As above, must not be used near animals, dangerous to operator (scalding)
Washing items in sinks or tubs	Inexpensive equipment	Labour intensive
Washing machines	Efficient, wide range of cycles	Machinery purchase and maintenance are expensive

[1] See Fig. 6.1.

some time to settle down once they have been put into new cages.

Once animals are removed from a cage the soiled bedding must be discarded before the cage can be washed. Emptying bedding from a cage causes a release of allergens and pathogens into the atmosphere creating a major risk to animals and staff. It is possible to utilise robotic systems to clean cages and so reduce exposure to harmful substances. However, the technology is in its infancy and it is very expensive to install. A more practical solution is to use cage cleaning stations which incorporate air extraction to contain allergens and pathogens (see Fig. 4.6).

Airborne allergens and pathogens are more difficult to contain when cleaning pens but vacuum cleaners fitted with high efficiency particulate air filters (HEPA filters) can be used to reduce the problem. In all situations staff involved with cage or pen cleaning should wear appropriate protective clothing.

Washing machines

After removal of bedding, cages need to be washed. Many types of machines are available for washing animal cages and ancillary equip-ment; they are usually either tunnel or cabinet washers.

Tunnel washers

A tunnel washer (Fig. 6.2) consists of a grid-type conveyor belt which carries cages through the tunnel past jets which spray hot washing solutions followed by rinse water onto all surfaces of the cages. The clean cages are unloaded from the other end of the machine. Larger types of tunnel washers provide pre-wash, acid wash (to remove scale) and hot air drying in addition to the main wash and rinsing sections. The spray jets are generally in fixed positions but are angled to ensure good coverage.

Cabinet washers

Cages are loaded onto special racks which are loaded into the machine (Fig. 6.3). The cages are washed by spray from moving jets on spinners or sliding batons. Some types have fixed jets that spray directly into the individual cages. To ensure efficient washing, materials must be loaded into the washer correctly. Numerous cycles of various temperatures, treatments and lengths can be se-

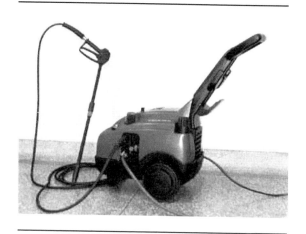

Fig. 6.1 High pressure hose.

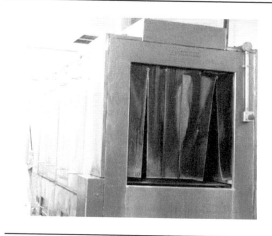

Fig. 6.2 Tunnel washer.

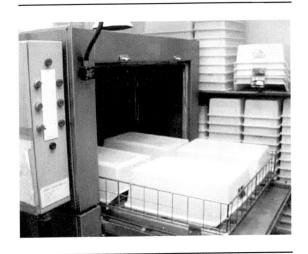

Fig. 6.3 Cabinet washer.

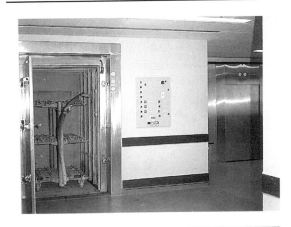

Fig. 6.4 Rack washer.

lected and some types also incorporate a hot air drying cycle. Cabinet washers are available in various sizes from small bench models up to large double-ended machines into which you can wheel large cage racks and primate cages.

Machines to wash animal water bottles and cage racks are generally of the cabinet design (Fig. 6.4) with both fixed and moving jets which inject wash and rinse solutions directly into each bottle.

The temperature and cleaning agents used in cage washers result in disinfected cages.

STERILISATION AND DISINFECTION

Although the physical removal of dirt will carry away vast numbers of micro-organisms and allergens, other more effective methods of destroying pathogenic organisms must be used regularly. These methods achieve either sterilisation or disinfection.

In order to work effectively the sterilisation or disinfection agent must come into direct contact with the organism it is intended to kill. Any dirt, organic matter or air that prevents this contact could allow organisms to survive the treatment, so cleaning must precede sterilisation or disinfection.

Sterilisation

Sterilisation is a process which results in the complete destruction or removal of all living organisms. Sterility is an absolute state; an area or object is either sterile or it is not. It cannot be nearly sterile.

Disinfection

Disinfection is a process that removes the causes of infectious disease. Disinfection does not destroy all forms of pathogenic organisms, it will not kill bacterial spores. The intention is to reduce the numbers of organisms to levels where there are too few to cause disease.

Pasteurisation

Pasteurisation is a form of disinfection that kills vegetative forms of bacteria by rapidly raising the temperature to 70° to 80°C followed by rapid cooling. The process is used to treat food because the times and temperatures used are effective in reducing micro-organisms but do not damage the nutrient quality. Pasteurisation was originally introduced to kill tubercle bacilli in milk. The pelleting process for laboratory animal diets achieves pasteurisation, reducing the numbers of viable micro-organisms in the diet from 5×10^6/g in raw ingredients to as little as 1×10^3/g in expanded pellets.

Fumigation

Fumigation is the use of gases or vapours in order to achieve disinfection.

METHODS USED TO ACHIEVE STERILISATION

Sterilisation can be achieved by the use of heat, chemicals, filtration and radiation.

Heat

Dry heat and wet heat are used.

Dry heat

Dry heat kills by coagulating or oxidising proteins. To ensure sterility materials must be exposed to very high temperatures for long periods. Dry heat has limited use in an animal facility because the material being treated is often damaged by the high temperatures. Dry heat methods include:

*   *Flaming* – In this method the material to be treated is exposed to a naked flame, either from a Bunsen burner or a flame gun. Temperatures of 500°C are reached with these techniques. There are obvious dangers with this method although it is often used to sterilise microbiological inoculation loops.
*   *Hot air ovens* – Metal or glass can be sterilised by exposure to temperatures of 160° to 180°C for one hour in hot air cabinets.
*   *Incinerators* – The most useful dry heat method of sterilisation is the incinerator. These are fuelled by gas or oil and are built to withstand temperatures in the region of 1000°C. At these temperatures a wide range of materials, e.g. carcasses, bedding and sharps, are reduced to an inert ash. Even highly infective materials are rendered sterile, although care must be taken when transporting infective material to the incinerator.

Wet heat

Wet heat destroys micro-organisms by denaturing proteins. The only effective method of achieving sterility uses steam produced above atmospheric pressure. Steam is an effective killing agent because of its specific heat of vaporisation and because it penetrates loads efficiently. In order to maintain steam under pressure a metal chamber called an autoclave is used.

Autoclaves are pressure vessels in which objects can be exposed to steam produced at above atmospheric pressure (Fig. 6.5). To work efficiently all air must be removed from the chamber. Two types of autoclave are used, the downward displacement autoclave and the pre-vacuum autoclave.

Downward displacement autoclave – In the downward displacement model, after the autoclave is loaded, steam is introduced from the top of the chamber. As steam is heavier than air it pushes the air out of the chamber through an exhaust valve at the base of the chamber. When a heat sensor in the exhaust registers the temperature of steam the valve is closed. It is assumed all the air has been pushed out and the chamber is full of steam.

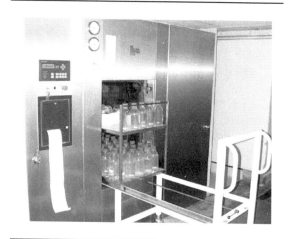

Fig. 6.5 Autoclave.

Downward displacement autoclaves are efficient for solid materials like cages, provided they have been loaded in such a way as to prevent air being trapped between them. Porous loads such as food are not sterilised in a downward displacement autoclave because it is impossible to get all of the air out of the load.

Pre-vacuum autoclave – Modern pre-vacuum autoclaves are able to cope with all types of loads. In these models a vacuum pump is fitted to withdraw air before steam is introduced. The air is removed and steam is introduced in a series of pulses (some air is sucked out and some steam is introduced, then more air is pumped out) until all the air is out and the chamber is full of steam. The vacuum ensures even penetration of steam throughout the chamber. At the end of the sterilisation cycle another vacuum is pulled which removes the steam which has the effect of drying the load.

Modern autoclaves are automatically controlled in order to make them more efficient and to prevent accidents due to human error. Each type of autoclave needs to be operated according to specific instructions and it is vital that these are strictly adhered to. It is also essential to load them properly to ensure even distribution of steam.

A wide variety of temperature, pressure and time cycles are available and the cycle should be selected that suits the type of material loaded in the chamber. Examples of appropriate autoclave cycles are:

- Polypropylene cages   121°C for 20 minutes
- Metal cages   134°C for 10 minutes
- Sawdust in steam   134°C for 25 minutes.
  permeable bags

Sterility will not be achieved unless the articles are packed and loaded in such a way that the stream is allowed to penetrate them.

Chemical sterilants

Very few chemicals are able to achieve sterilisation. The few that do are toxic and should only be used in controlled conditions. An example of a chemical sterilant is peracetic acid which is used as a surface sterilant for isolators and their supplies. In addition to its high toxicity it is unstable and easily inactivated. Other, less toxic, chemicals are superseding this agent.

Filtration

Micro-organisms can be removed from air and liquids by trapping them in filters.

Radiation

Ionising radiation emitted in the form of gamma rays (usually from a cobalt[60] source) is an effective sterilising agent. Exposure has to be done at specialist units because the process is very dangerous and requires expensive installations. The rays destroy organisms by damaging DNA. Many materials used in animal units are treated with gamma radiation, e.g. food, bedding, hypodermic syringes.

Ultra-violet radiation will also achieve sterilisation but as these rays have very poor penetration ability they can only be used for surfaces or very thin layers of material.

METHODS USED TO ACHIEVE DISINFECTION

An ideal disinfectant should be:

- Lethal to the undesirable micro-organisms and should not permit the establishment of resistant forms.
- Harmless to animals and to man (e.g. non-toxic, non-irritant, non-allergenic, non-corrosive).
- Harmless to materials (e.g. non-corrosive, non-staining).
- Not inactivated by the presence of materials, especially organic matter.
- Quick to work at a wide range of temperatures.
- Compatible with other chemicals, e.g. detergents.
- Suitable for a wide range of applications.
- Easy to use with good powers of penetration.
- Easily stored with a long shelf life.
- Reasonably priced at use dilution.

No disinfectant has all of the above properties; for instance, no disinfectant process can be relied on to destroy bacterial spores and all are inactivated by organic matter to some extent.

Disinfection can be achieved by the application of heat and chemical means.

Heat

Heating methods that can be used to disinfect:

- Boiling water or steam at atmospheric pressure (free steam) can be used to reduce the numbers of micro-organisms on materials.
- Immersion in boiling water exposes materials to temperatures not exceeding 100°C. It is useful to treat water and heat resistant materials like surgical instruments.
- Steam lances – can be used to treat exposed surfaces.
- Steam chests – caging and equipment can be treated in a steam chest which is either an enclosed box containing boiling water over which the equipment is suspended or a box into which steam is supplied. Exposure times of approximately 1 hour are necessary to achieve adequate disinfection.

Chemical disinfectants

Routine chemical disinfection is used in all animal units. It is important to be aware of the limitations of disinfectants; they should only be used in the way the manufacturers advise. Disinfectants must be freshly made up when used and excess disinfectant should be discarded in an approved manner after use. All utensils used to apply the disinfectant should be cleaned after use, preferably with a different type of disinfectant. This prevents the establishment of resistant strains of micro-organisms (that is strains of micro-organisms that are able to survive exposure to the disinfectant).

The properties and use of some of the major groups of disinfectants are given below. This should only be used as an illustration of the different agents available. Within most groups there are

many disinfectants, each with different activity. Before using any agent the manufacturer's literature should be consulted.

Phenols and derivatives

Properties: These agents are bactericidal, fungicidal and destroy some types of viruses (enveloped viruses) but have no effect on bacterial spores. Their activity is reduced by the presence of organic material and oils. They are more active in an acid pH and also when in hot solution. They are stable at use dilution which is usually 1 to 2% and have fair rinsing properties. Phenolic compounds are toxic, corrosive and have an unpleasant smell. They should not be used in areas housing cats and dogs as these species are particularly sensitive to them.
Uses: Application to surfaces, e.g. walls and floors, following the removal of gross soiling.

Alcohols

Properties: These are bactericidal, fungicidal and virucidal but have no effect on bacterial spores. They are readily inactivated by organic material and oil. Normal use dilution is 70% but they are not stable due to vaporisation (absolute alcohol has no disinfectant properties).
Uses: They are used to treat clinical thermometers and clean surgical instruments. They are particularly useful for wiping clean surfaces and sensitive equipment, e.g. electronic balances and hair clippers, as the vaporisation brings about rapid drying. They are incorporated in detergents for skin disinfection.

Formaldehyde

Properties: This agent is bactericidal, bacteriostatic, sporicidal, fungicidal and virucidal, being more active in hot solution. Use dilution can vary from 1 to 40% depending on method of use but the stability is poor. It is a highly toxic chemical and should only be used for fumigation in controlled conditions.
Uses: Fumigation (used at 40%).

Iodophors

Properties: Iodophors are bactericidal, sporicidal, fungicidal and virucidal. Activity is enhanced by an acid pH and heat. They have low toxicity but have poor rinsing properties. Use dilution is usually 1 to 2% and at this concentration they are stable.

Uses: Skin disinfection. Footbaths and dunk tanks. Clean surfaces.

Chlorine, e.g. sodium hypochlorite

Properties: Bactericidal, sporicidal, fungicidal and virucidal. Activity is reduced by a factor of 10 for every unit of pH above 7. Increasing temperature increases activity but temperatures in excess of 500°C may cause the liberation of free chlorine. They have low toxicity but are corrosive because they are oxidation agents. They have good rinsing properties but are not very stable at use dilution which is normally 1 to 5%.

Uses: Water treatment. Feeding and watering utensils and animal cages and ancillary equipment when combined with a compatible detergent. Chlorinated detergents can be used in cage washing machines.

Quaternary ammonium compounds

Properties: Selectively bactericidal and bacteriostatic. Some compounds are also fungicidal and virucidal. Good detergency. Activity can be reduced by anionic and non-ionic detergents, hard water, rubber and plastics, oil and some metals.

Activity is enhanced by an alkaline pH and heat. They are stable at use dilution which is usually 1 to 2%. They have low toxicity and poor rinsing properties due to surface adsorption. Such compounds contain cationic detergents which can remove fat from the skin. Numerous different types of quaternary ammonium compounds are commercially available for use as disinfectants and the level of activity will vary considerably between different types.

Uses: Treating surfaces, e.g. walls, floors and bench tops following the removal of gross soiling. Feeding and watering utensils followed by thorough rinsing. Combined with compatible detergent in cage washing machines. Skin disinfection at low concentration.

Amphoterics (ampholytic surface active agents)

Properties: Fungicidal and selectively bactericidal and bacteriostatic. Good detergency. Activity is reduced by the presence of organic material, anionic and non-ionic detergents. Activity is enhanced by heat. Rinsing properties are poor due to their surface activity but they leave an active residue behind which can be advantageous in certain situations. They have low toxicity but the detergency properties can cause removal of fat from the skin. Stable at use dilution which is normally 1 to 2%.

Uses: Surfaces following the removal of gross soiling, particularly when it is advantageous for an active residue to remain. Skin disinfection at low concentration.

Chapter 7
Feeding and Watering

FOOD

In nature, animals manage to fulfil their nutritional requirements by eating a variety of foodstuffs. In the animal house they only have the diets provided for them. In theory animals eat to satisfy their energy requirements, which implies that when these are satisfied the animals stop eating even if they have not taken in enough of the other nutrients. It is, therefore, necessary to ensure that laboratory animal diets contain the nutrients they require in the proportions that will satisfy their needs.

The nutrients that must be present in the diet of an animal are proteins, fats, energy sources (which can come from carbohydrates, proteins or fats), vitamins and minerals. In addition to these nutrients food often contains undigestible fibre which provides no nutrient value but is a necessary aid to efficient digestion.

The amount of each nutrient required by an animal depends on several factors:

- Its physiological condition (growing, pregnant and lactating animals have a high demand for nutrients).
- Its activity (active working animals require more energy than inactive ones).
- Its age (old animals tend to need different amounts of nutrients than younger ones).
- Its species (some species have a specific requirement for a particular nutrient, e.g. primates and guinea pigs for vitamin C).

The amount of food consumed by the animal will be affected by the above but the following factors will also have an influence:

- Palatability.
- Physical form (hard, soft, powder).
- Boredom (a few species such as cats and primates may get bored with a diet and may stop eating it; many species eat more because they are bored and have nothing else to do).

In addition to formulating diets for individual species laboratory animal diet manufacturers provide diets for specific purposes, for instance:

- *Maintenance diets* – provide the nutrients necessary to keep an animal in good condition, neither gaining nor losing weight
- *Breeding diets* – provide the extra nutrients required to support pregnancy, lactation and growth
- *Autoclavable diets* – include supplements to make up for those lost in the high temperatures of an autoclave.

PRESENTATION OF DIET

In the wild most species find their food on the ground. In captivity, in order to keep the food clean and to try to prevent wastage, diet is normally presented in containers. A variety of containers are used to accommodate the animals' feeding behaviour and the type of food they eat.

Bowls are used for animals that are likely to eat a whole ration immediately after it is presented

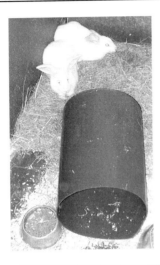

Fig. 7.1 Food bowl in floor pen.

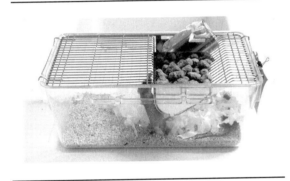

Fig. 7.2 Mouse cage showing food basket.

(e.g. dogs), where mashes or seeds are fed or when animals are housed in pens (Fig. 7.1). Baskets or hoppers are used where the animal eats little and often and when the food is intended to last for several days (e.g. rabbits and rodents) (Figs 7.2, 7.3). The shape and size of the food container used will be affected by the species, the size and age of the animal (and therefore the amount they consume) and the number of animals in the cage or pen. Where more than one animal is housed in a cage, food should be presented over a wide area; animals are competitive feeders and some dominant

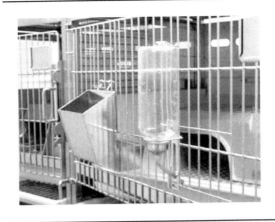

Fig. 7.3 Rabbit hopper and water bottle.

individuals will try to prevent others in the cage from feeding. The wider the area of food presentation the less successful they will be.

The Latin term *ad libitum* (*ad lib*) which means 'at one's pleasure' is used to describe the practice when food or water is freely available to an animal at all times. The term restricted feeding is used when food is only available for part of the day.

Forms of diets

Food is presented in different physical forms to suit the requirements of the animal and experimental demands.

Pelleted diets

Diets are pelleted to reduce waste and to make them easier to handle. The ingredients are ground and thoroughly mixed during manufacture to produce a homogenous mixture so the animals cannot selectively eat individual components.

Two types of pellet are produced, traditional and expanded (Fig. 7.4). Traditional pellets are produced by mixing and grinding raw materials with steam. The mixture is then passed through a pelleter, under mechanical pressure, and it emerges from the die face as pencil shaped pellets.

Raw materials for expanded pellets are mixed

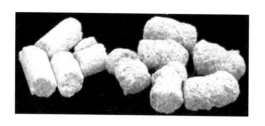

Fig. 7.4 Traditional pellets (left) and expanded pellets (right).

in the same way but additional steam is introduced into the pelleting machine (called an expander) as the mixture is passing through. This causes a build-up of temperature and pressure within the expander. When the pellets emerge from the die into atmospheric pressure the compressed steam they contain expands producing the larger pellet. The higher temperature reached in expanders 'cooks' the ingredients, producing a harder biscuit-like texture.

Expanded diets are more attractive to animals and cause less waste although they take up more space in the hopper.

Powdered diets

Powdered diet consists of finely ground components. The usual method of manufacture is to pass diet that has already been pelleted through a grinder. This ensures that the quality of the diet is similar to the 'normal' pellets and that the particle size is consistent. Powdered diet is especially useful when experimental work requires test substances to be added to the diet.

Mash

Mash consists of powdered diet mixed with water. The diet is readily eaten when in this form. However the increased water content encourages rancidity and mould growth so fresh mash must be made up immediately before feeding and changed at least daily. In view of this and the fact that the containers in which the mash is fed must be fre-

quently cleaned, feeding mash is very labour intensive. Mash can be used to feed sick or weak animals and is a particularly useful method to supply food to some transgenic strains.

Mixed feeding

Some animals, e.g. primates, benefit from being fed with pelleted diets and supplementary fresh natural foods.

ASCORBIC ACID (VITAMIN C)

Ascorbic acid provides an illustration of a specific nutrient requirement of some animals. Primates (including humans) and guinea pigs are unusual in that they cannot synthesise vitamin C in their tissues, therefore it must be included in their diet. As it is a water-soluble vitamin it is not stored in the body, so it must be fed every day.

A deficiency of vitamin C (commonly known as scurvy) in the guinea pig will first show as a staring coat and a reluctance to move. A severe case might show loose teeth, bleeding gums, haemorrhages under the skin, stiff and swollen joints, the long bones may break easily and death may follow.

Vitamin C is easily converted into an inactive chemical when exposed to oxygen; oxidation is speeded up if it is hot or in the presence of some metals.

Methods of administration of vitamin C

Traditionally there have been three methods of ensuring primates and guinea pigs obtain sufficient amounts of the vitamin. In practice, feeding supplemented pellets is the only one routinely used, although fresh fruit is fed to primates to make the diet more interesting and ascorbic acid can be added to water in emergency or for experimental reasons.

Incorporated in a pelleted diet

Diet manufacturers incorporate vitamin C supplement during the pelleting process. Extra supplement is added to diet that is intended to be autoclaved before feeding.

Advantages All animals consume the vitamin C while taking in other nutrients. No extra labour is required.

Disadvantages There is a possibility of oxidation losses, but provided the diet is used before its use-by date this should not be a problem. Only diet with extra vitamin C supplementation should be autoclaved.

Supplemented in drinking water

This may be in the form of a soluble tablet or powder of ascorbic acid or as a fruit juice supplement for primates.

Advantages Administration is totally under the control of the person looking after the animal.

Disadvantages Labour intensive as the water bottles have to be removed, emptied and refilled each day to ensure that sufficient vitamin C is available. One animal may drink its share and waste the rest – this is particularly characteristic of the behaviour of guinea pigs.

Vitamin C breaks down on contact with metal drinking spouts – this can be overcome by the use of plastic tops; however, these may be chewed by guinea pigs. Monkeys tend to drink several mouthfuls at one time and thus obtain sufficient vitamin C from the bottle as the contact with the metal spout has not been for a sufficient length of time for it to have been broken down.

Supplemented by means of fresh fruit and/or vegetables

For example, guinea pigs – cabbage, primates – fresh fruit and vegetables.

Advantages Animals derive pleasure from consuming such supplements. Extra feeding improves man-animal relationships and gives an extra opportunity to observe the animals in movement. The vitamin C content does not deteriorate quickly if good storage is maintained.

Disadvantages The vitamin content of vegetables is variable and cannot be guaranteed. Relatively large quantities of fruit and vegetables may have to be stored in proper conditions. There is a risk of microbial contamination, e.g. with *Pasteurella* or *Salmonella*. Washing, cutting and feeding the diet is labour intensive. Grouped animals may not all get a fair share of the supplement as one or two may 'hog' what is available. This could be overcome by deliberately overfeeding but any uneaten surplus will increase the smell and may make cage cleaning more difficult. A costly means of providing ascorbic acid.

This method is valuable for the variation it gives to the diet of animals, particularly primates. It can only be used for animals in conventional units.

DIETS FOR LABORATORY ANIMALS

Mice, rats and Syrian hamsters

Mice, rats and hamsters will all do well on laboratory rodent diet. There are a variety of diets commercially available. The ingredients in a typical rat and mouse maintenance diet are shown in Table 7.1. Rodents are normally fed pelleted diets in basket-type hoppers.

Rabbits and guinea pigs

There are many different pelleted diets available for rabbits and guinea pigs. Examples of the ingre-

Table 7.1 Rat and mouse diet.

Ingredients	% composition
Cereal products	88.5
Wheat	
Barley	
Wheatfeed	
Proteins	8.5
Extracted soya bean meal	
Whey powder	
Energy sources	0.5
Soya oil	
Supplementation	2.5
Vitamins	
Major minerals	
Trace minerals	
Amino acids	

Table 7.2 Guinea pig diet.

Ingredients	% composition
Cereal products	49.75
Wheat	
Oats	
Barley	
Wheatfeed	
Proteins	17.5
Expeller linseed cake	
Fish meal	
Fibre sources	30.0
Grass meal	
Supplementation	2.75
Vitamins	
Major minerals	
Trace minerals	

Table 7.3 Standard rabbit diet.

Ingredients	% composition
Cereal products	39.0
Barley	
Wheatfeed	
Proteins	13.5
Extracted soya bean meal	
Whey powder	
Energy sources	0.5
Soya oil	
Fibre sources	45.0
Wheat bran	
Oat by-product	
Grass meal	
Supplementation	2.0
Vitamins	
Major minerals	
Trace minerals	
Amino acids	

dients of a typical guinea pig diet and rabbit diet are shown in Tables 7.2 and 7.3.

Diets for rabbits and guinea pigs have a considerably higher fibre content than rat and mouse diets. Rabbits and guinea pigs are usually fed from hoppers.

Ferrets

Ferrets survive well in laboratories when fed on commercial cat or dog pellets. Tinned cat or dog meat can also be fed. They are usually fed from open bowls.

Dogs

A complete dry diet may be fed *ad libitum* or as a daily measured ration in accordance with the recommendations of the manufacturer. This will constitute a balanced diet if fed together with unrestricted water. Dogs may also be fed traditional dog biscuits with cooked or tinned meat. It is usual to feed dogs from open bowls.

Cats

A complete dry food for cats may be fed *ad libitum*. It is very important to ensure that abundant water is always available when feeding a dry diet. Cats can also be fed proprietary tinned cat food but care should be taken in selecting the brand as quality varies. It is usual to feed cats from open bowls.

Rhesus monkeys

Several commercial pelleted diets are available for these Old World monkeys. Although such diets are fortified with vitamin C during manufacture, it is still recommended that the diet is supplemented with fresh fruit and/or vegetables as the animals obviously enjoy consuming natural foods and the

Table 7.4 Average amounts of dry diet and water that might be offered to a fit, adult male per day.

	Diet (g)	Water (cm³)
Mouse	5	6
Rat	15	35
Syrian hamster	10	8
Guinea pig (800 g)	40	100
Rabbit (3 kg)	150	500
Ferret	65	45
Cat (3 kg)	200	500
Dog (12 kg)	400	1500
Macaque (per kg body weight)	50	75

Note: The above figures are given as a guide. Many factors influence the amount an animal eats and drinks. Certain animals will be wasteful, particularly with water, and should therefore be offered more.

variety reduces the boredom that can occur with the same pelleted diet and provides environmental enrichment. Average amounts of dry diet and water that might be offered to adult male animals per day are listed in Table 7.4.

DIET QUALITY

Diet quality depends on the ingredients used, the manufacturing process and the conditions the diet is kept in between manufacture and being eaten by the animal. Diet that has been properly manufactured, cooled and packaged may still be contaminated during manufacturer's storage, delivery and in diet storerooms and bins on users' premises. Prior to use, diet should be kept in cool, dark, dry, well-ventilated conditions that are insect and vermin proofed in order to protect the diet from chemical deterioration, spoilage and contamination by organisms.

Chemical deterioration

Natural interactions between the chemical components of the foodstuffs occur at a rate that depends largely on the temperature. An ambient temperature of less than 15°C will reduce this problem to an acceptable level. Sunlight causes a rise in temperature and increases the rate of oxidation of the food. This affects the vitamins

and the fats, which become rancid causing a reduction in the palatability and nutritional value of the diet.

Spoilage and contamination by organisms

Temperatures above 15°C increase the metabolic and proliferation rates of organisms that may spoil the food. All such organisms require a source of water and their activities are limited by low relative humidity. Both temperature and humidity are limited by adequate ventilation. Dark conditions tend to discourage many of the flying insects. Details of some of the organisms that cause the deterioration of diet are given later in this section.

If spoilt or contaminated food is fed to animals, there is a danger that it will no longer meet their nutritional requirements and contamination from outside sources could give rise to poisoning or infectious diseases.

Storage of diet

Diet stores should be cool, dry, dark, well-ventilated, insect and vermin-proofed and easily cleaned.

The diet should be stacked on pallets or duck boards to ensure good circulation of air and to avoid condensation (Fig. 7.5). Walls of storerooms should be free from cracks and crevices and should not be penetrated by pipework, so there are no places for insects to hide.

Uninsulated hot water or steam pipes should not pass through diet stores. Rodent barriers should be fitted to doors, and fly screens should be fitted to openings. The use of insect electrocutors may be advantageous.

Foodstore management

Food stores should contain only food.

On receipt, all bags should be checked and any showing signs of dampness, damage or discoloration should be rejected. Open bags should not be kept in the diet store. Care should be taken when handling diet bags within the store so that the risk of damage to bags and the diet within

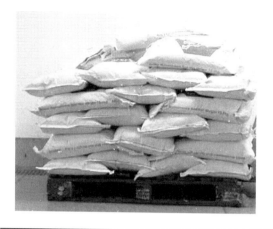

Fig. 7.5 Diet stored on a pallet.

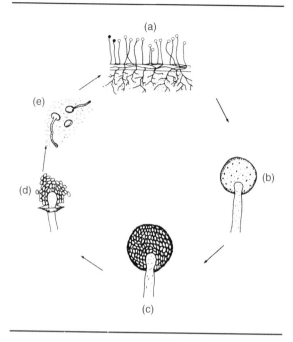

Fig. 7.6 Life cycle of typical mould. Clockwise from top: (a) mould with hyphae growing into the food and aerial hyphae bearing spores; (b) developing spores; (c) ripe spores; (d) spores being released; (e) released spores germinating.

them is minimised. Any spillage should be cleaned up immediately. Diet should be stacked to facilitate use in strict rotation, i.e. oldest diet first. Diet should always be used before the expiry date.

The amount of diet taken from the store should be strictly limited to the immediate requirements as the food storage conditions within the animal rooms are not ideal. Diet bins or other food containers should be routinely emptied and cleaned. Bins and feeding hoppers should not be continually topped up as the diet at the bottom may remain for long periods and deteriorate. Empty diet bags should be removed from the area as the food dust they contain can attract food pests.

Food stores should be regularly cleaned and inspected for signs of infestations.

ORGANISMS CAUSING DETERIORATION OF DIET

Although detail of the life history of food pests is included here for interest, the most important requirement is to be able to recognise the *signs* of infestation. The species described here represent a small sample of the pests that could be found in a food store.

Moulds

The spores of moulds are ubiquitous; they grow quickly in warm, moist conditions (Fig. 7.6). Many types may affect foodstuffs, e.g. pin mould and mildews. The presence of moulds may be clearly seen if they are well established but may be recognised earlier by a musty smell.

Dry conditions from manufacture to use will normally eliminate the problem. Most moulds only cause food spoilage but some will also cause respiratory disease in animals and humans if inhaled. The mould *Aspergillus flavus*, commonly found on the groundnut, produces aflatoxin that can be fatal.

Arachnids

The only arachnids that infest foodstuffs are mites, one example of which is the flour mite.

Flour mite

Adult females are 0.5 mm long whilst the males are slightly smaller at 0.4 mm (Fig. 7.7). The body is translucent, white and sparsely covered with hair; the legs are pale violet. The adult mites have four pairs of legs but the larvae have only three pairs.

Mass infestation by flour mites only occurs in damp conditions. The female lays about 20 eggs that hatch into white larvae about 0.15 mm in length. These six-legged larvae then pass through two eight-legged nymph stages before becoming adults.

As the adults are so small it is difficult to detect them in the diet. In the case of a severe infestation the mites will appear as a moving layer of dust. Infestation by mites leads not only to damage caused by their feeding, but also produces a bad smell and causes rapid deterioration of the foodstuffs.

Insects

Many insect pests may infest or contaminate foods, including flies, cockroaches, crickets, moths, silverfish, beetles and weevils. Infestation by insects is not necessarily harmful to the nutritional value of the diet but it could indicate that patho-gens have been introduced and that the diet should not be fed to the animals.

Flour moth

The body of the adult moth is approximately 13 mm long with a wingspan of 20–25 mm (Figs 7.8, 7.9). The forewings are blue-grey with dark wavy transverse bars and a row of dark spots at the tip. The hind wings are pale grey. During the day the moths usually cling to ceilings and walls and they usually fly about at dusk. Mating takes place immediately after the adults emerge from the co-coon and up to 350 eggs are laid during the first four days. The eggs are laid in a sticky secretion in or near the diet and hatch 3–17 days later. The caterpillars are whitish with a reddish-brown

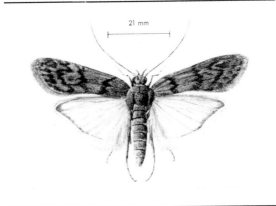

Fig. 7.8 Flour moth.

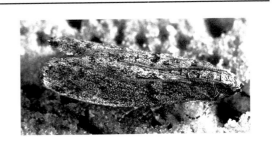

Fig. 7.9 Flour moth with closed wings.

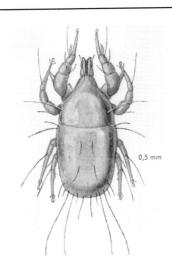

Fig. 7.7 Flour mite.

head. A silken thread is produced from a gland near the mouth and trails of this thread are left behind in the diet, giving the appearance of webbing. After three to five moults the caterpillars are full-grown and 15 to 19 mm long. They eventually find a corner or crevice in which they spin cocoons and pupate for 7–16 days. These moths overwinter as caterpillars but, in contrast to other species, usually remain in the foodstuff.

As with most moths, it is the caterpillars that do the damage. The food is contaminated with excreta and silk thread.

Grain weevil

The adults are 3–5 mm long and dark brown, nearly black in colour (Fig. 7.10). The head ends in a slightly curved proboscis and the neck shield has depressed markings and is almost as long as the longitudinally grooved wing covers.

The female lays up to 200 eggs at a rate of 2–3 per day depending on temperature and humidity. Each egg is placed in a small hole bored in the pelleted diet or grain and sealed with a mucilaginous plug of saliva. The eggs hatch into larvae in 8–11 days to give small, white, legless larvae that feed within the diet. The larvae moult four times and finally pupate within the diet after 6–8 weeks. After a further 5–16 days the adult weevil bores its way out of the diet and infestation of the diet will only be apparent at this stage. The full life-cycle takes about six months. The weevils cannot fly.

Infestation will cause a reduction in the quality and weight of the pellets and they will be tainted with white, dusty excreta which contaminate the diet as well as rendering it unpalatable. The diet will be heated which accelerates the development of the weevils and the diet will be liable to cake and mould. Temperatures may be attained which actually kill the insects.

Saw-toothed grain beetle

The adult beetles are 2.5–3.5 mm in length (Fig. 7.11). The body is dark brown with two deep longitudinal grooves and six pointed projections on either side of the pro-thorax (hence the name 'saw-toothed').

The female lays up to 400 eggs, either singly or in small batches, at a rate of 6–10 per day. The eggs are laid in, or adjacent to, a suitable food supply and hatch after 8–17 days. The larvae are flattened and yellowish-white with brown flecks and a brown head. They are freely mobile and grow through a series of moults from 0.9–3 mm in length. The larvae feed on the damaged food, so they can be regarded as secondary pests of diet. The larval stage lasts from 4–7 weeks and they construct a cell of diet particles and other debris in which to pupate. The adults emerge after 1–3 weeks.

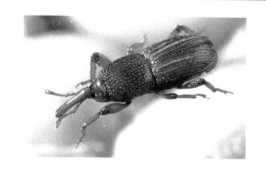

Fig. 7.10 Grain weevil.

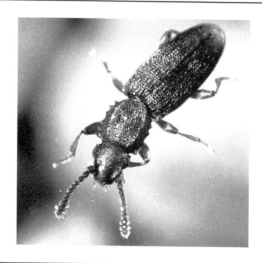

Fig. 7.11 Saw-toothed grain beetle.

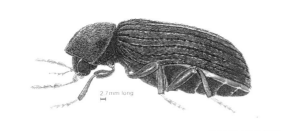

Fig. 7.12 Biscuit beetle.

These beetles physically damage the diet and, when infestation is heavy, will heat the diet. Both the quality and weight of the pellets may be reduced and the palatability severely affected.

Biscuit beetle

The adult beetle is 2–4 mm in length. It is reddish-brown in colour with short yellowish fine hairs covering its body (Fig. 7.12). The female lays about 100 eggs singly within or around the diet over a period of about three weeks. The eggs hatch after 1–2 weeks to produce very small, active larvae that wander about the diet and may even penetrate packaging to infest the diet within. Over a period of 2–5 months the larvae undergo four moults to achieve a full-grown length of 5 mm. At this size the larvae are incapable of movement and construct cells of food particles and saliva in which to pupate. Although the pupal stage lasts for 9–18 days, the adults may remain in the cocoons for up to two weeks before emerging. The adult beetles live for up to eight weeks but do not feed. Badly infested diet will be full of small round holes and tainted with the excreta of the larvae.

Cockroaches

German cockroach or steam fly (Fig. 7.13) – The adults are approximately 12 mm long. The female produces 4–8 egg capsules at approximately one month intervals. Each thick-walled resistant capsule is about 6 mm long and contains up to 30 eggs. The female carries the capsule for 2.5–4 weeks until just before the eggs hatch. The capsules are

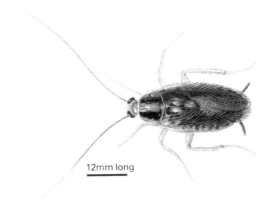

Fig. 7.13 German cockroach.

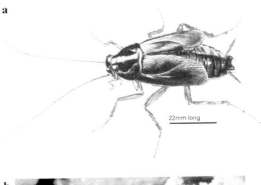

a

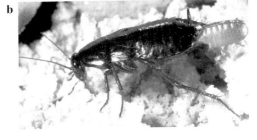

b

Fig. 7.14 a Oriental cockroach. **b** Oriental cockroach with egg sac.

usually concealed near to a food source and the nymphs pass through 5–7 moults between hatching and gaining maturity.

Oriental cockroach (Fig. 7.14) – The adults are approximately 22 mm long. The female produces five egg capsules at monthly intervals. The thick-

walled resistant capsules are 12 mm in length and
contain up to 16 eggs. The capsules are cemented
to the substrate in the vicinity of a food supply and
may be covered in debris. Nymphs emerge 8–12
weeks later and progress through 7–10 moults
before reaching maturity, which may take up to
two years depending on conditions.

Cockroaches are potential vectors of disease
and can contaminate animal diets as well as the
animals themselves. Good hygiene will go a long
way in the control of cockroaches.

Housefly

The adults are 5–6 mm long with a wingspan of
13–15 mm (Fig. 7.15). The thorax is grey with four
longitudinal dark stripes. The basal half of the
abdomen is buff coloured and occasionally trans-
parent at the sides with a central dark band.

The female commences egg laying two days
after emergence as an adult. During her adult life
of 1–3 months she is capable of producing 4–5
batches of 100–150 eggs. The pearly-white cylin-
drical eggs, 1 mm in length, are laid in moist decay-
ing matter. The eggs hatch in 8–48 hours, giving
smooth, white legless maggot larvae. The larvae
bury away from light and after three moults reach

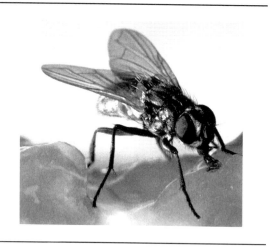

Fig. 7.15 Housefly.

maturity at a length of 10–12 mm. Mature larvae
go in search of cool surrounding areas and develop as yellow, brown or black pupae 5 mm long.
Adults emerge from three days to four weeks later
depending on temperature.

Houseflies can transmit many disease-causing
organisms including intestinal worms and their
eggs. They will frequent and feed indiscriminately
on any liquifiable solid food, which could be moist
putrefying material, animal waste products or
food stored for human or animal consumption.
Flies liquify food by regurgitating digestive juices
and stomach contents on to the food substance.
This 'liquid' is then drawn up by the suctorial
mouth parts together with any pathogenic organisms that are present. These collect in and on their
bodies to be transferred to other food or survive
passage through the gut to be deposited as fly
spots.

WATER

Water is an essential part of the diet of animals;
50–70% of an animal's body consists of water.
It is the medium in which most chemical reactions
take place within the body, it lubricates the movement of limbs and organs, supports tissues and is
the medium which transports materials around
the body. A little water is also used up in chemical
reactions. Cooling of the body takes place because
of the heat energy used up in evaporating water
from the body surfaces, particularly from the
lungs and mouth and, in some species, through
sweating.

This vital need for water should be met by
making water constantly available to animals. In
most circumstances, water suitable for human
consumption is adequate for laboratory animals,
i.e. water direct from the main supply. This water
is referred to as being 'potable'. However, water
from the mains supply is not sterile. Water treatment works reduce the level of organisms in the
water to levels that will not cause disease. If
the water from this source is allowed to stand
in tanks, bottles or other containers before it is
used the few micro-organisms that remain in it
may reproduce to levels where they do present
a disease risk. It is important, therefore, to ensure

water fed to laboratory animals is directly from a mains supply.

In full barrier units water may need to be further treated to ensure it is sterile. This can be done in a variety of ways, e.g. by adding acid or chlorine, by passing it through an ultra violet light source, by ultra filtration or by autoclaving.

Methods of presenting drinking water

The methods of presentation vary according to the drinking habits of the species and the volumes consumed. Experimental design and work routines can also affect the method used. Suitable methods of presenting water to each species are given in Table 7.5.

Open bowls

All animals can drink naturally from open bowls, though most are inclined to make a mess. Water in the bowl can be soiled or spilt, making the cage and the animal wet. Small animals may be at risk of drowning. Wherever possible the bowls should be fixed to prevent overturning. Even so they will need cleaning and refilling at least twice a day. For these reasons bowls are not widely used; however, they are the most suitable method for cats and are sometimes used for dogs. Reducing the amount of open water in the cage limits wastage, contamination and mess.

Bottles

A spout (sipper tube) attached to an upturned bottle, which acts as a reservoir, ensures water is constantly available (see Fig. 7.3) but limits the opportunity for contamination and wastage.

The system only provides the correct water supply if the orifice of the spout is of sufficient size to allow free flow when used by the animal, but is small enough to prevent air entering the tube when it is not being used. The mechanics are such that an animal cannot drink from a completely full bottle, and nearly empty bottles will empty themselves. Simple ball valves in the tube may prevent the latter problem and may also reduce wastage caused by the animal shaking the bottle (Fig 7.16). Spouts must be inspected for wear and limescale build up.

The amount of water provided to any cage or pen depends on the species and the number and size of the animals that occupy it. Two smaller bottles are better than one large one because if one large bottle leaks, the animals are left with no water and a flooded cage. If one smaller bottle runs out, a supply of water is still available, the flooding is limited and two bottles ensure that a dominant animal cannot stop cage mates from drinking.

Water bottle systems are initially cheaper to purchase than automatic systems but are more labour intensive to maintain.

Table 7.5 Suitable methods of presenting water to each species. The choice of system depends on many factors including the cage design and the experimental requirements.

	Open bowl	Bottle and spout	Automatic valve
Mouse	—	•	•
Rat	—	•	•
Hamster	—	•	•
Guinea pig	•	•	•
Rabbit	—	•	•
Ferret	•	•	•
Cat	•	—	—
Dog	•	—	•

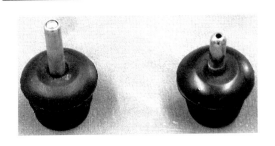

Fig. 7.16 Water bottle drinkers – the one on the left has a ball valve.

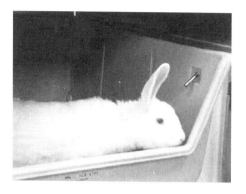

Fig. 7.17 Automatic water drinker.

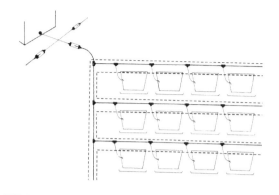

Fig. 7.18 Automatic watering system.

Automatic piped systems using valves

Two types of valve, in various sizes, have been developed for use in a piped water supply. The toggle-type is more often used in pens with drainage, whereas the spring-loaded types with washers are generally used in boxes.

Valves can be mounted directly onto cages in any position or fixed permanently to the rack or wall so that they project through holes in the backs of cages (Fig. 17.17). This allows cages to be removed for cleaning without disturbing the drinking system.

Usually, the valves within each room are fed from a tank through fixed or flexible pipes (Fig. 7.18). The tank is fed through a ball cock from the mains. Periodically the system is flushed to ensure stale water does not collect in the pipes. The tank and pipe work should be accessible for inspection and cleaning.

Automatic systems are expensive to install and their cleaning is time consuming. Automatic systems still have to be checked daily to ensure that the valves are supplying water to the animals. It is impossible to know if the animal is drinking or how much the animal is drinking. Leaking valves can cause considerable flooding.

Chapter 8
Breeding Common Laboratory Animals

EXPLANATION OF BREEDING TERMS

Species
: A group of organisms showing close similarity in physical characteristics.

Colony
: A group of animals of the same species kept together for a particular purpose.

Closed colony
: A colony that does not take in any animals from outside, all new stock is bred from within.

Strain
: A group of animals with known ancestry, usually with some distinguishing characteristic.

Inbreeding
: Mating of close relatives.

Inbred strain
: A strain that has been produced as a result of 20 consecutive generations of brother × sister matings or youngest parent × offspring matings. Inbred strains are useful for some types of research because the results of the experiments are not affected by genetic variation. Inbred strains are often weaker than non-inbred strains. They have smaller litters and are more susceptible to disease and environmental stress. Inbred strains have to be bred by monogamous pairs and very careful breeding records have to be kept to ensure the colony remains inbred.

Genetically modified
: Animals that have been altered by the addition or subtraction of genetic material by the use of genetic engineering techniques.

Transgenic animals
: Animals that have had genetic material from another species introduced into them by genetic engineering techniques.

Knock out
: Animals that have some genetic material removed from their genome by genetic engineering techniques.

Knock in
: Animals that have extra genetic material added to their genome by genetic engineering techniques.

Outbreeding
: The deliberate avoidance of inbreeding. Selecting animals for breeding that are not related. This produces the widest possible genetic diversity within a colony.

Random breeding
: Selecting animals for mating without any regard to their relationship. To be strictly random animals should be selected using random number tables or a random number generator. Some of the breeding animals may be related, others will not, at each generation the situation will change.

Oestrous cycle
: The reproductive cycle in the female mammal. It is described as having four stages: pro-

oestrus, oestrus, met-oestrus and di-oestrus. The stages reflect the changes that occur in the female body so that she will mate, ovulate, provide a site for the egg to be fertilised and a place for the developing young to be nourished and grow.

Oestrus
The stage in the oestrous cycle when the female will allow herself to be mated (called 'heat' in some species). Mating occurs near to ovulation so that sperm is available to fertilise the egg when it is shed.

Post-partum oestrus
The oestrus that occurs very soon after giving birth in some species. If males are with the females during birth they will mate and so shorten the litter interval.

Ovulation
Release of eggs from the ovary. In some species ovulation is *spontaneous* where it occurs regularly after each oestrus. In other species it is *induced*, that is stimulated by mating.

Fertilisation
The union of the male and female gametes (eggs and sperm) to form a zygote.

Implantation
Embedding of the zygote into the lining of the uterus.

Delayed implantation
If a female is under great physiological demand (e.g. if she is rearing a large litter) implantation may not happen immediately. It can be delayed for about five days.

Placenta
An organ derived partly from maternal tissue and partly from embryonic tissue which attaches the embryo to the uterus and through which nutrients and gases pass to the developing animal and waste products are removed.

Mating, copulation, coitus
Intromission of the penis into the vagina so that male gametes can be deposited to enable them to fuse with the female gametes.

Age at first mating
The age at which animals are first paired for mating. This is usually later than the time at which the animals are first capable of becoming pregnant.

Gestation period
The period between fertilisation and parturition.

Pseudo-pregnancy
Outward signs of pregnancy in a female when fertilisation has not taken place. It may be caused by sterile matings or it may occur when mating has not occurred at all. In most species it lasts for about one half to two-thirds of the normal gestation period. In the ferret and bitch it is of the same duration as the gestation period. In the bitch it may follow an unsuccessful mating or can occur even if the bitch has not been mated.

Embryo
Name given to developing young in the early stages of pregnancy.

Foetus
Name given to developing young from the time they become recognisable.

Parturition
The process of giving birth.

Breeding season
The period in the year when animals that do not breed continuously come into breeding condition so that they mate and become pregnant.

Lactation
Production of milk.

Fostering
Rearing of young by females other than their own mothers.

Cross fostering
Technique where young are taken from a number of mothers and resorted in some way (e.g. same sex or same number) before being reallocated to females for rearing.

Weaning
Gradual change in diet of young animals from milk to solid food. Completion of weaning is often forced when animals are removed from the parent's cage.

Pre-weaning mortality rate	The number of young dying between birth and weaning expressed as a percentage of the number born.
Economic breeding life	The time during which an animal is producing litters of sufficient quality and quantity so that it is more cost effective to continue to breed from it than to replace it with new breeding stock.
Timed mating, dated mating	Mating arranged so that young will be born on a known day, i.e. mating may be observed or identified by the presence of copulatory plugs or when females are known to be in oestrus.
Culling	Removal of weak, old, sick or excess stock from a colony.

BREEDING SYSTEMS

The term breeding system refers to arrangements made in order to produce animals of the desired type. It includes arrangements for mating, husbandry of parents and offspring, replacement of breeding stock and provision of special requirements such as solid floored caging, nesting material, nest boxes, whelping quarters etc.

Criteria for the choice of system

In order to breed laboratory animals successfully a system has to be devised that takes into account the behaviour and reproductive physiology of the animal and the desired characteristics of the young produced.

Examples of the effects of reproductive physiology

Although all the animals covered in this chapter have an oestrous cycle there are differences between them which need to be taken into account when devising a breeding system. Some females are able to mate all year round (e.g. mice and rats) while others only mate at certain times of the year, in the breeding season (e.g. ferrets). In most seasonal breeders it is the female that has a definite breeding season; the male is able to mate all year.

In the ferret the male is only sexually active during the breeding season. Some animals ovulate at a set time in each reproductive cycle (spontaneous ovulators), in others mating stimulates ovulation (induced ovulators).

Examples of the effects of behaviour

Behaviour can affect breeding systems in a variety of ways, for instance, female rabbits object to males being present when giving birth in confined spaces. Syrian hamsters will fight if put together for the first time when adult, unless the female is in oestrus when they will mate. Females of many strains of rats object to other females being present during birth.

Desired characteristics

Animals may be required with specific genetic characteristics, which determines the type of breeding system that must be used, for instance the primary line of an inbred strain must be bred using monogamous pairs. In other cases there may be a request for no specific genetic type, in which case harems may be the most appropriate system as they are cheapest to operate.

Mating arrangements

Monogamous pairs

Housing one male and one female together, usually throughout their breeding lives. The young remain with the parents until weaned. This method is expensive because it requires more space, labour and materials and requires as many males as females. However, it does take advantage of postpartum oestrus, pre-weaning losses are low and accurate record keeping is straightforward.

Harems

Housing one male with two or more females. Harems can be permanent where the males and females remain together throughout their breeding lives, or non-permanent (or boxing out system) where the females are removed for parturition and returned to the harem when the young are weaned.

In permanent harems young remain in the harem until they are removed when weaned. Fewer males are required and the method is less expensive on space and maintenance than monogamous pairs; in addition post-partum oestrus can be taken advantage of. Accurate breeding records are more difficult to keep because females may have litters at the same time and the females of some species share feeding and rearing duties.

Boxing out is used where it is necessary for the parentage of young to be accurately recorded or in those species who do not like to give birth in the presence of others (e.g. rats). Post-partum mating cannot be used in this system but there tends to be lower pre-weaning loss because there are fewer animals in the cage and less competition for milk.

Arranged mating or hand mating

A selected female in oestrus is taken to a male's cage or pen for mating. She is either left for a period of time or until mating is observed, and she is then returned to her own cage. Detailed records may be easily kept. The system is expensive on space and labour.

Breeding records

Records must be kept in order to ensure the colony continues to produce quality young from identifiable parents in an economic way. In order to keep full records, animals must be individually identified.

The information recorded is determined by the breeding system used and the particular demands on the colony. Ideally, data should be recorded so that the ancestry of each animal can be traced back to the origin of the colony.

The information required for full records for each breeding animal is as follows:

- Identity.
- Parentage.
- Date of birth.
- Date(s) of mating and/or pairing.
- Identity(ies) of mate(s) used.
- Cause of death.

and for each litter would be:

- The parentage.
- Date(s) of mating or pairing.
- Number in litter at birth.
- Sex of litter at birth.
- Causes of any deaths.
- Number in litter at weaning.
- Sex of young at weaning.
- Weight of young at weaning.
- Date of weaning.
- Fate of offspring.

Standard forms are usually devised to record breeding performance. Cards are often used so that they may be filed for easy reference. On all forms a space should be available to record the physical condition, behaviour and fate of the offspring.

A modern alternative to written records is records stored on computers. Programs are available that will store and analyse breeding records on a continuous basis.

Selection of breeding stock

In random breeding systems the selection is by random numbers.

In other systems breeding stock are selected from the information available in their records and from the appearance of the individuals. Delaying selection until the second or subsequent litters from a female enables more information about her breeding performance to be available and therefore more reliable decisions to be made.

The ideal future breeding animal would be:

- Free from visible (or detectable) unwanted abnormalities or characteristics.
- From 'good litters' in terms of:
  - number of offspring
  - size of offspring
  - even sex distribution
  - acceptable litter interval.
- From parents with good previous records.
- From parents of good temperament and good 'mothering' ability.

When finally selecting breeders, particular attention should be paid to the condition of the genitalia (e.g. well developed testicles in males, clean appearance to the vulva in females) and to characteristics such as the appropriate number and arrangement of teats.

Breeding systems for each species

The mouse

In the proximity of the male, the unmated female has an oestrous cycle of four or five days. The length of oestrous cycle tends to increase in the absence of the male. Obvious external signs of oestrus are difficult to detect by humans. The type of breeding system implemented must therefore leave the detection of oestrus to the male by giving him ready access to the female so that mating can take place. The phase of oestrus lasts for about 12 hours and usually occurs at night.

Mice are usually bred from monogamous pairs or in permanent harems as the males tend not to interfere with the young and females co-operate in feeding and rearing the young. It is usually unnecessary to box out females or to foster litters. Keeping mice in permanent pairs or harems enables advantage to be taken of post-partum oestrus. If this oestrus is missed the oestrous cycle recommences after lactation.

Matings are usually only arranged when known birth dates are required. In this case oestrus can be detected by taking a smear from the vagina (vaginal smear), and observing it under the microscope for the detection of cells characteristic of oestrus. Alternatively the vagina can be inspected on the morning following pairing for the presence of a cream coloured, waxy substance known as a copulation plug (Fig. 8.1). The plug only remains in the vagina for a few hours before falling out and it indicates that mating has taken place.

Gestation usually lasts 19–21 days but, when frequent successful post-partum matings occur, the gestation period may lengthen by as much as five or six days due to delayed implantation. Young mice are removed from the parents' cage at 19–21 days to same sex groups. This ensures they are removed before the arrival of the next litter.

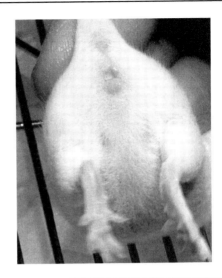

Fig. 8.1 Vaginal plug in female mouse.

The rat

The oestrous cycle in the rat takes 4–5 days to complete. Oestrus lasts approximately 12 hours and usually occurs at night, but mating may be observed during the day.

Rats can be bred in monogamous pairs or harems. It is usual practice to box out pregnant females as their intolerance of the presence of others when rearing young results in high pre-weaning mortality. The vaginal plugs of rats are easily seen but are more likely to have fallen out by the next morning. So if timed matings are required the rats can be kept in grid bottomed cages for mating with paper on the tray underneath the cage so the plugs can be easily seen.

Gestation lasts for about 21 days. Parturition usually takes place in the early morning. Weaning and the recurrence of oestrus after mating is the same as for mice.

The Syrian hamster

The unmated female has an oestrous cycle of about 4 days. If it is necessary oestrus can be identified by observing the presence of a cream

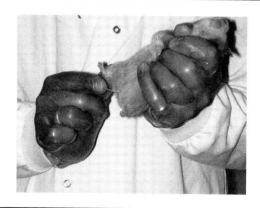

Fig. 8.2 Post ovulatory discharge in hamster.

coloured, stringy discharge, with a distinctive smell from the vagina (Fig. 8.2). This is the post-ovulatory discharge and signals the end of oestrus. The next oestrus will occur three days after the discharge is noted. If the female's back is stroked she will raise her tail and arch her back (behaviour known as 'lordosis') when she is in oestrus. Oestrus lasts for approximately 12 hours. Copulation plugs are not seen.

Syrian hamsters can be bred from harems or monogamous pairs providing they are set up at weaning age. If it is necessary to mate adult hamsters, arranged mating must be used. In this case the female is taken to the male's cage and mating observed. If mating does not occur the female may act aggressively to the male and must be removed immediately. As hamsters are most sexually active just after dark, the room lighting can be adjusted so darkness occurs during the working day.

The hamster has the shortest gestation period of the common laboratory animals – 16 days. Post-partum oestrus occurs but mating is unlikely to be successful at this time. The oestrous cycle will resume at the end of lactation. The young are weaned by 21 days.

A minimum of 12 hours of light and temperatures of 21°C will prevent hamsters from hibernating in winter and minimise seasonal effect on the breeding performance.

The guinea pig

The guinea pig has an oestrous cycle which lasts for 14 days and oestrus lasts 24 hours. Female guinea pigs have a hymen (a membrane across the vaginal opening) which regresses spontaneously a day or two before oestrus and regrows after each oestrus.

Guinea pigs are usually bred from permanent harems with a ratio of up to 1 male to 10 females. As the gestation period is long and the lactation is short, post-partum mating is not likely to be detrimental. Young guinea pigs will often feed off other lactating females. Boxing out of pregnant animals from a harem, breeding in monogamous pairs or arranged matings are usually only implemented when specifically required.

Mating takes place during day or night and is, therefore, more often observed than in the other small species. Copulation plugs do occur but are fairly difficult to find. After the long gestation period of 65–72 days, the young are well developed at birth and consequently the lactation period is short at about 14 days. Oestrus will recur post-partum and again at the end of lactation.

The rabbit

Oestrus lasts for several days, for several weeks or until the female is mated. The readiness of the female to mate is indicated by a reddened and slightly enlarged vulva. Due to the antagonism of the doe to the buck when kept in confined conditions rabbits are only bred from arranged, observed matings. The doe is taken to the buck, mating is observed and the animals are separated. Ovulation is induced by mating and it is advisable to repeat the mating on the next day to ensure successful fertilisation.

The gestation period of large breeds such as New Zealand White is 30 days; smaller breeds such as Dutch have gestation periods of 28 days. Rabbits have a post-partum oestrus but remating at this time is not recommended. The female shows signs of oestrus again at about the fourth or fifth week of lactation.

When parturition is imminent, the doe will strip the fur from her underbody to supplement the nesting material supplied in the nest box or nesting area. In addition to providing a comfortable nest this allows the young to feed with greater ease and it enables heat to be transferred to the young more readily. It is advisable not to interfere with very young litters as rabbits tend to reject or even kill their young if they are handled. Does only feed their young once a day. Weaning is complete at between five and eight weeks.

Although there is no definite breeding season there will still be a considerable reduction in production in the autumn and winter months in spite of any environmental control.

The ferret

Ferrets are usually bred from arranged, observed matings.

The vulva of the female is grossly enlarged and red to purple in colour when she is in oestrus. Both male and female ferrets have a definite breeding season and sexual activity only occurs during the period from March to July, although the season may be extended by the alteration of lighting regimes (early or late wintering). Oestrus is prolonged in the absence of the male and ovulation is induced by mating.

During courtship and mating the male drags the female around the pen. Tying occurs and mating may be prolonged. The gestation period is 42 days. Oestrus will recur at the end of lactation if it is still within the breeding season, hence it is possible to get two litters from a female ferret in one year. Weaning is complete between six and eight weeks.

The cat

Cats are seasonal breeders in natural light conditions but will breed all year round providing they are exposed to 12–14 hours' light a day. They have an oestrous cycle of 14–21 days and oestrus lasts for 3–10 days. Cats are induced ovulators. They are bred by arranged mating or in large harems.

A female in oestrus is easy to recognise from her wailing, rolling and the arching of her back (lordosis). With arranged matings the female is taken to the male and they are left together for 24–48 hours.

During mating the male grips the female around her body and grips her neck with his teeth. Mating is rapid, one thrusting movement stimulates ejaculation. At the end of mating, as the male withdraws his penis, the queen gives a loud shriek and exhibits post-mating behaviour pattern which involves rolling and licking her vulva. Humans or toms who attempt to approach her during this time risk being attacked. After 20–30 minutes the tom will be allowed to come near and the mating process will be repeated. The sensation caused by the withdrawal of the penis provides the stimulus to induce ovulation.

The gestation period lasts for just over nine weeks and the females are boxed out into a littering cage about one week before parturition. The young are fully weaned by 6–8 weeks.

Oestrus will usually recur during the fourth week of lactation.

The dog

Pro-oestrus may be detected by observing a blood stained discharge from the vulva. The vulva swells and the discharge becomes straw coloured as the bitch enters oestrus. Oestrus occurs about 10 days after the first discharge is noted. Where arranged matings are used, it is usual to mate the animals on three alternate days. At oestrus the bitches will 'stand' for mating.

Dogs are unusual in that they have no seminal vesicles and in order that the semen should be effective, secretion from the prostate gland (which provides the medium for the sperm to swim in) is produced after the ejaculation of the sperm. This apparently necessary secretion takes place over a period of time when the animals are tied together. This tying results from the swelling of a glandular portion of the penis within the vagina.

The normal oestrous cycle of the bitch is about 6–7 months long. Pregnancy has little effect on the cycle. More bitches come into oestrus (season or heat) in the spring and autumn than do in the summer and winter. The gestation period lasts for 9–10 weeks.

WEANING

In small rodents (mice, rats and Syrian hamsters) it is usual to complete weaning by removing the young from their dam on a specific day according to a routine. This is done at about 3 weeks but, with inbred strains that exhibit poor growth, weaning may be delayed if the female is not pregnant.

Guinea pigs are often weaned when they achieve a certain bodyweight, e.g. 180–200 g (at about 14 days of age). Rabbits are usually weaned by age, at 6–8 weeks. Ferrets, cats and dogs are also usually weaned at between 6 and 8 weeks of age but each litter is usually treated as individuals.

Pre-weaning mortality

The reproductive mechanism is not faultless and a small percentage of deformed, small or unthrifty animals (runts) will occur in any colony but may not be seen as parents often eat such young. These runts, and some offspring which are born apparently normal, may not survive until weaning due to disease, poor mothering, competition for food or deficiency in the nest or the general environment.

An awareness of any increase in the pre-weaning mortality rate of a breeding colony is a valuable aid to the early detection of problems.

Economic breeding life

In the smaller laboratory species it is usual to replace breeding stock as follows:

- Rats, mice and hamsters   after about 6 litters
- Guinea pigs   after 6–8 litters
- Rabbits   after 10–12 litters or, in a small colony, depending on the breeding performance of individuals.

Although the breeding performance of males does not diminish at the same rate as that of females, it is usual, in the smaller species, to replace the males at the same intervals as the females.

In the larger laboratory species, e.g. ferret, cat and dog, the economic breeding life will depend on the breeding performance of the individual animals. With these carnivores, it is usual to replace the male long before his breeding life is over in order to prevent him from inbreeding with his own daughters.

Productivity

The productivity of a particular female is usually assessed by the number of offspring weaned per week (or month or year). Such calculations are influenced by the sizes of the litters at weaning and the interval between litters.

The table in Appendix 1 shows the expected average litter intervals, litter sizes and productivity of the common laboratory species, but variation is likely to be encountered between different strains and colonies.

Chapter 9
The Physical Development of
Young Animals

Mice and rats

Mice and rats are born into well-formed nests (Plate 1). They are naked and their eyelids are closed but they are able to move sufficiently to find a teat and can squeak to attract the attention of their mother. Communication between mother and young is often in ultra sound. The ages of mice and rats may be estimated from their physical development. Table 9.1 details stages of development in average outbred strains of mice and rats. Considerable variations occur between different strains of animals, for instance Wistar rats are smaller than Sprague Dawley rats and inbred CBA mice are larger than inbred DBA mice. Inbred strains will not only be smaller than outbred but develop at a slower rate.

These variations should be noted when interpreting Table 9.1 and other tables and charts in this book.

Syrian hamsters

Like mice and rats Syrian hamsters are born into well-formed nests. Their physical development is similar to that of the mouse.

Guinea pigs

Guinea pigs do not make proper nests, as the young are well-developed when born. At birth they are already covered with short fur, eyelids are open and they are capable of eating solid food, although the female provides milk for 14 days.

They are fully mobile within a few hours and have the appearance of small adults within 14 days of birth.

Rabbits

Rabbits construct nests with any material available to them; the doe lines the nest with fur taken from her abdomen. Unless absolutely necessary, young should not be disturbed until they start to leave the nest at about 2–3 weeks of age. The female may reject young that have been touched. The kits are born hairless, with their eyes closed, but are able to move a little for feeding. By seven days they have doubled their birth weight, have a well-developed coat and are able to move more easily. By ten days the eyes are open and the ears are functioning (Plate 5). Between 15 and 21 days they leave the nest and feed independently. Weaning is completed between five and eight weeks.

The carnivores (ferrets, cats and dogs)

A nest area is normally provided for these species. The young are born with fur but with eyelids closed. They can crawl to find a teat and can vocalise to attract their mother's attention. The eyelids open at about two weeks. Young are totally dependent on milk for about the first four weeks of life and will eat soft solids before learning to lap. They are all usually weaned between six and eight weeks of age (Plates 6, 7).

Table 9.1 Stages of physical development in outbred mice and rats.

New-born	The eyelids are closed. Pups are naked except for short whiskers. They appear bright pink with translucent skin, which enables the abdominal organs to be seen. If the pup has suckled, the milk is visible in the stomach. The earflaps (pinna) are small and are tight to the snub-nosed head (Plate 2).
2–3 days	Whiskers are longer and more obvious. The skin is a duller pink and opaque and the internal organs are no longer as visible. The pinna start to lift away from the sides of the head.
About 5 days	Coloured strains begin to show skin pigmentation.
8–10 days	Most of the body is covered by short, fine fur of its final colour.
About 10 days	The incisors erupt and the teats of young females become obvious because they are not covered by fur (Plate 3).
12–14 days	Eyelids are open. The snout is longer and pups are very mobile when disturbed.
14–16 days	They are well covered with fur. They spend more time out of the nest and begin to eat the crumbs of diet below the hopper.
17–18 days	The pinna are larger and stand away from the head. Fur fully covers the underbelly.
19–23 days	The first and second pair of molars erupt and at this stage the pups are self-sufficient and weaning can be completed (Plate 4)
Mice at 5 weeks and rats at 7 weeks	The young reach sexual maturity, the vagina is open and the testes have descended into the scrotal sacs. The third pair of molars erupt.

Table 9.2 Approximate ages and weights at different stages of development.

Species	Birth weight	Weaning age	Weaning weight		Age at first mating	Weight at first mating	Adult body weight
Outbred mice	1–1.5 g	19–21 days	10–12 g	M	6 weeks	20 g	45 g
				F	6 weeks	20 g	40 g
Outbred rats	4–7 g	19–21 days	40–60 g	M	12 weeks	200 g	800 g
				F	10–11 weeks	150 g	600 g
Syrian hamsters	1.5–2.5 g	21 days	35–45 g	M	6 weeks	80 g	120 g
				F	6 weeks	80 g	130 g
Outbred guinea pigs	50–100 g[1]	14 days	180–200 g	M	4 months	500 g	1 kg
				F	3 months	450 g	800 g
Dutch rabbits	30–50 g	5–8 weeks	300–500 g	M	8 months	2.5 kg	3.5 kg
				F	6 months	2.0 kg	2.5 kg
New Zealand white rabbits	60–80 g	5–8 weeks	1–1.5 kg	M	9–10 months	3–3.5 kg	6 kg
				F	7–8 months	2.5–3 kg	5 kg
Ferrets	10 g	6–8 weeks	300–400 g	M	12 months[2]	700–800 g	1–2 kg[4]
				F	9–12 months[3]	700–800 g	0.85–1 kg
Cats	120 g	6–8 weeks	0.5–1 kg	M	12 months	3 kg	5 kg
				F	9 months	2.5 kg	3.5 kg
Dog (Beagle)	400 g	6–8 weeks	1–1.5 kg	M	18 months	12 kg	14–16 kg
				F	14 months[5]	10–12 kg	10–12 kg

[1] Dependent on litter size.
[2] First season.
[3] First season.
[4] There is a marked seasonal weight variation with both sexes.
[5] Second oestrus.

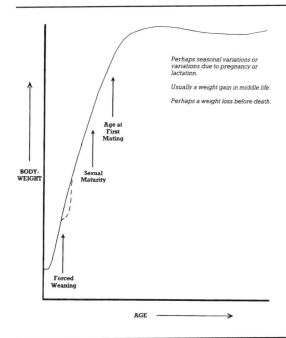

Perhaps seasonal variations or variations due to pregnancy or lactation.

Usually a weight gain in middle life.

Perhaps a weight loss before death.

Age at First Mating

Sexual Maturity

BODY-WEIGHT

Forced Weaning

AGE

Immediately following birth there is likely to be a small weight decrease which should soon be replaced as suckling becomes more effective. There is then a rapid increase in weight through the primary growth phase followed by a probable slight check at weaning.

Sexual maturity is usually reached before the rapid growth phase begins to slow down. It is usual to wait until the animal has nearly attained full size before trying to breed from it so that it is more physically able to withstand the strains and stresses of pregnancy and lactation.

The age at puberty and hence the age at first mating for males is usually a little later than those for females in order to be sure of effective mating.

Adult males tend to be about 10% heavier than females of the same age.

Fig. 9.1 Typical growth curve.

DEVELOPMENTAL DATA

Table 9.2 details the timing and weights of each species at key stages of their development. Figure 9.1 shows the typical pattern of growth in a young mammal.

Chapter 10
Identification of Animals

Individual animals must be identified so that accurate records can be kept of their experimental and/or breeding history. The Animals (Scientific Procedures) Act 1986 requires all animals to be identified. In the case of dogs, cats and primates, the method used must be permanent and approved by an inspector.

Some animals may have more than one form of identification, for instance a dog may have a tattoo bearing its litter and personal number and a collar and disc that can be read without having to handle the animal.

CHARACTERISTICS OF AN IDEAL METHOD

An ideal method of identification should be:

- *Harmless to the animal* – The method should be painless when applied and comfortable for the animal to wear. It should cause no subsequent discomfort through irritation, constriction, infection or toxic effect.
- *Simple to apply and maintain* – The method should require no great skill and should be able to be applied quickly. It should require no maintenance once applied.
- *Easy to read and decipher* – The method should be able to be read without having to handle the animal. If a code is used it should be simple to decipher by anyone including the Home Office Inspector.
- *Sufficiently permanent* – In many cases animals

must carry identification for life but on occasions the requirement is for a much shorter period.
- *Compatible with other requirements* – Whatever method is used it must not interfere with other activities; an ear tag would not be suitable for a rabbit that was to be bled from an ear vein, or colour code marking for a guinea pig that was being used for a skin test.

Unfortunately there is no single method that is ideal. Most permanent methods cause momentary pain and care must be taken to minimise this with the appropriate use of analgesics. Rapid application by skilled technicians will reduce discomfort felt by the animal. Invasive techniques should only be used when non-invasive ones are inappropriate.

Factors which influence the choice of identification method

The method selected to identify animals is influenced by a variety of factors among which are:

- Species, age/size, colour, temperament or behaviour of animals.
- Number of individuals concerned.
- Experimental conditions.
- Availability of equipment and skills.
- Cost.

METHODS OF IDENTIFICATION

Describing the physical characteristics of animals

Animals that show variation in appearance (e.g. beagles, cats, hooded rats and multicoloured guinea pigs) can be identified from a written description, diagram or a photograph recording distinguishing characteristics (sex, coat colour distribution, build). The method is only efficient for small numbers of animals due to the limited variation in the animals and to the time required to decipher them.

Applying stains

Coloured markers can be used to stain the fur or tail skin of light-coloured animals. The method is only suitable for temporary identification because it will wear off quickly. If longer term identification is required, the marking has to be repeated at least every 10 days (Fig. 10.1).

Marking can be done with histology stains or felt or fibre-tipped pens containing non-water-soluble ink. The solvent for the ink must be checked to ensure it will not harm the animals (particularly very young ones) or affect experimental results. Histology stains are applied with cotton buds or with a fine paint brush. Examples of stains that can be used are:

- Red – acid, basic or Carbol Fuchsin
- Violet – gentian, methyl or crystal violet
- Green – brilliant, ethyl or malachite green

These are all usually used at 1–5% weight/volume solution in 70% alcohol.

Marker pens are available in a wider range of colours; those commonly used are red, blue, green and black.

Stains should be applied in small patches and be worked well into the fur. It is important to ensure that stains are dry before replacing animals in their groups.

Codes for this method are only easy to learn for fairly small numbers of animals. The code must be displayed where the animals are housed or used. Staff with colour blindness may have difficulty interpreting the marks.

Ear and toe punching

Small pieces of the pinnae of rats and mice can be removed in a coded pattern using a small hole punch or scissors (Fig. 10.2). The technique requires a lot of skill in order to minimise the discomfort to the animal and to avoid mistakes (which cannot be rectified once made). The code must be devised so that a minimum number of ear pieces are removed. A complicated code results in very delicate ears that may tear easily; it is also very difficult to decipher.

The ear punch can be used on most strains of animals as it is not affected by skin colour. However, it is not the most appropriate method for aggressive strains as these may tear ears when fighting. A few strains (such as those on a SCID background) regenerate tissue, closing the hole or notch.

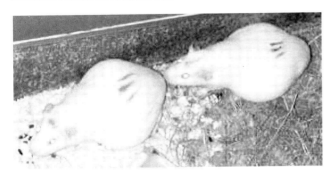

Fig. 10.1 Identification stains on guinea pigs.

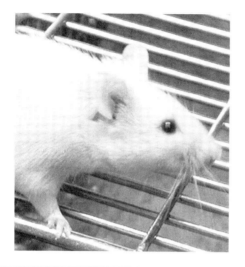

Fig. 10.2 Mouse with punched ear.

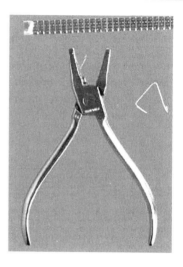

Fig. 10.3 Ketchum tag.

Toe punching is carried out on chickens by punching holes through the web between the toes, according to a predetermined code.

Fixing studs and tags to ears

A variety of studs and tags are available to fit most sizes of animals from small rodent to large farm animals. They are made from metal, soft plastic and hard plastic. Some are self piercing whilst others require a hole to be punched first. They can be colour coded as well as being numbered which allows for the identification of both groups and individuals.

Tags are available in two main types, ketchum tags and rototags. Ketchum tags enclose part of the outer edge of the ear and must be placed with care or the ear may grow around them (Figs 10.3, 10.4). Alternatively if too much room is allowed for growth the animal may catch the tag and pull it out. Rototags and studs do not have this problem as they do not enclose the ear (Fig. 10.5).

Small animals will have to be handled in order to read an ear tag.

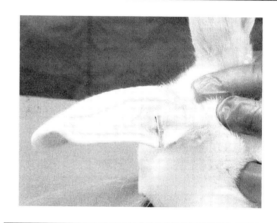

Fig. 10.4 Ketchum tag in ear of a rabbit.

Tattooing

Tattooing is a technique that introduces dyes into the dermal layer of the skin. If applied properly it is permanent, although the ink may leach into surrounding tissue making the tattoo indistinct over time (Fig. 10.6).

There are two methods of applying the tattoo, with pliers (Fig. 10.7) or with a tattooing pen. Both

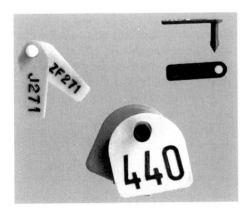

Fig. 10.5 Rototags.

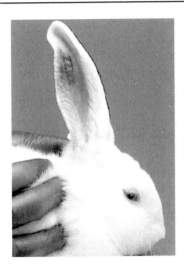

Fig. 10.6 Ear tattoo.

methods require skill to produce a clear tattoo and to minimise the discomfort caused to the animal. Tattoo ink is available in white and green as well as black, so dark-skinned animals can be tattooed.

Pliers hold interchangeable pin punch tattoo numbers or letters. Sterile pin numbers or letters

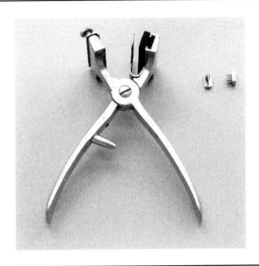

Fig. 10.7 Tattoo pliers.

are loaded into the pliers and the number is punched into a sheet of paper to ensure it is the correct one (mistakes cannot be corrected). The ear is cleaned, disinfected and may have local anaesthetic rubbed on; it is held between the jaws of the pliers so that the pins are in contact with the inner surface of the ear. The jaws are firmly closed. Tattoo ink is then rubbed over the surface of the ear where it will enter the puncture wounds. Excess ink is rubbed off.

An electric tattoo pen has a vibrating needle which can be used to write the identification code freehand.

Rings or bands

The use of leg rings is restricted to rabbits and birds. Leg rings are available in two forms: closed rings consisting of a continuous band of material, and split (or adjustable) rings. Rings can be colour coded or bear numbers or text. The method is non-invasive but the animal has to be handled for the ring to be read (Figs 10.8, 10.9).

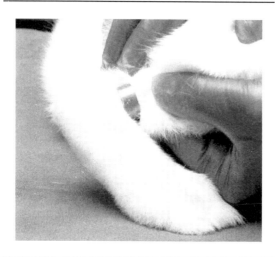

Fig. 10.8 Rabbit leg ring.

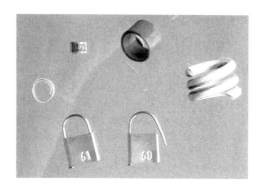

Fig. 10.9 Chicken wing tags and leg rings.

Rabbits

Solid rings are available from the British Rabbit Council and are sized for each breed. Such rings are rarely used in the laboratory as they are permanent and have to be fitted when the rabbit is young. Adjustable leg rings are more commonly used; these are applied just above the hock joint. Numbered leg rings must be frequently checked as, when the rabbit grows, the ring becomes tight causing damage to the tissue.

Birds

Closed rings for birds are species specific. The correct sized ring must be slipped over the foot of the young bird (normally at approximately 7 days old). The foot of the young bird is lubricated, the three forward toes are placed into the ring and it is slipped over the ball of the foot and up the leg until the hind toe is free of the ring. Once the leg and foot achieves its full size the closed ring will not slide off over the foot. Split rings may be applied to the bird at any stage in its life.

Applying tags or clips to wings

Chicks can be easily identified by the use of wing clips. The safety-pin type is easily inserted but is readily lost, and the Ketchum tag is permanent. Both require some skill and experience in insertion as they must be placed through the web of the wing and not through the muscle (see Fig. 10.9).

Adult birds which are being handled regularly may be easily identified by a numbered, coloured plastic wing tag which is attached by a press stud or a band that is slipped over the wing.

Collars and chains

Neck collars with discs can be used for cats and dogs. The collar must be loose enough to allow the animal to escape if it becomes caught, so these can only be used as a back up to a permanent method of identification.

Collars and discs are available in a number of colours and the disc can hold a variety of information. They must be fitted with room for growth and must be checked and adjusted regularly, as often as once a week in rapidly growing animals.

Chains and discs secured around the neck or waist can be used with marmosets but there is always a risk of the animal becoming tangled in the cage furniture (Fig. 10.10).

Electronic tagging

Electronic tags are transponders (microchips) which can be programmed with an alphanumeric system allowing up to 54 billion different identifi-

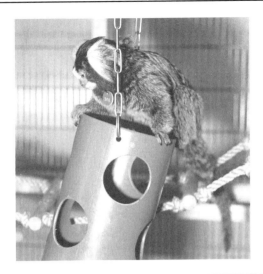

Fig. 10.10 Marmoset wearing identification collar.

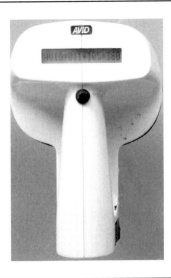

Fig. 10.12 Transponder reader.

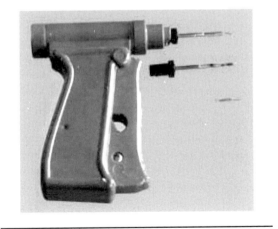

Fig. 10.11 Transponder applicator – showing needle and transponder.

cation codes. The transponder is activated by a radio-wave emitted by a reader (Figs 10.11, 10.12); when the reader receives and processes the code it displays it on a liquid crystal display. Alternatively it can be downloaded into a computer. Some systems can be read up to 1 m away from the animal.

The transponder is inserted subcutaneously using a purpose designed applicator fitted with a large hypodermic needle. There is little or no tissue reaction but some transponders migrate away from the site they were deposited in.

Implanting the transponder is not a regulated procedure. However, some types are available that measure physiological parameters, such as body temperature, as well as providing an identification code. Implantation of these devices is a regulated procedure.

Chapter 11
Experimental Procedures

Experimental procedures are concerned with the administration of substances and collection of tissues and body fluids. This chapter explains some of the terms and describes some of the techniques used in experimental procedures. It is not intended to be a practical guide. Techniques described here should only be performed by a suitably trained person. Experimental procedures are regulated by the Animals (Scientific Procedures) Act 1986 (see Chapter 12). Those carrying them out on protected animals must hold a personal licence and must be working under the authority of a project licence at a designated scientific procedure establishment.

All techniques mentioned here are demonstrated in the IAT video *Procedures with Care*.

ADMINISTRATION OF EXPERIMENTAL SUBSTANCES

The basis of many animal experiments is to administer a test substance to an animal and observe reactions to it. The ways in which test substances are administered are similar to the ways in which medicaments are given to treat disease. There are many routes by which substances could be administered to an animal, the choice of route being dependent on the species of animal, the nature of the substance and experimental considerations.

Routes of administration

Enteral routes

This involves administration of substances into the alimentary canal where they can be absorbed into the blood stream through the gut wall.

Example – oral routes (or *per os*) means via the mouth. Three main methods are used:

- Dietary   Inclusion of test substance in food or water.
- Capsule   Test substance is placed into a gelatine capsule which is placed at the back of the animal's mouth and swallowing is induced by stroking the throat; capsules are tasteless and easily swallowed.
- Gavage   The word means 'forced feeding' and refers to techniques whereby test substances are administered by means of a tube, connected to a syringe (Fig. 11.1). The animal is suitably restrained and a tube is passed to the back of the mouth; when the animal swallows, the tube enters the oesophagus and may be advanced to the stomach where the substance can be slowly injected. Care must be taken to ensure the tube does not pass into the trachea.

Enteral routes also include substances administered via the rectum. This route is not often used but some substances are readily absorbed by this route.

Parenteral routes

Routes of administration other than by introduc-

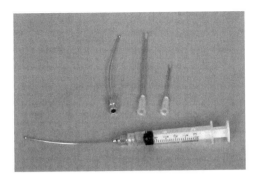

Fig. 11.1 Oral dosing equipment.

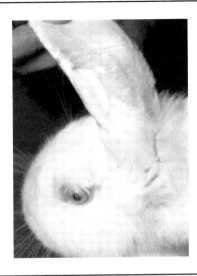

Fig. 11.2 Local anaesthetic over marginal ear vein prior to introducing hypodermic needle.

tion into the alimentary canal. They are either by topical application or by introduction into the body by other means.

Topical routes – applying substances directly onto the surface of the region of the body which is to be affected by them:

- Dermal or cutaneous Application of liquids, creams or pastes on to the skin.
- Intranasal Insertion of drops into the nose.
- Intraoccular Insertion of drops into the eye.
- Inhalation Inspiration of gases, vapours or aerosols into the lungs.

Other parenteral routes – these techniques usually require administration by means of a hypodermic needle. An exception to this is percutaneous.

- Percutaneous Application of a substance to the skin in a form that will be absorbed into the body tissues.
- Intradermal Injection of substance into the layers of the skin.
- Subcutaneous Injecting substances into the layer of connective tissue immediately under the skin (a common site is the scruff of the neck).
- Intramuscular Injection of a substance into a muscle (large muscles in the thigh are usually used; care must be taken to avoid blood vessels, nerves and bone).
- Intraperitoneal Injection into the peritoneal cavity (the space between the abdominal wall and the abdominal organs); the injection is made near the midline halfway between the lowest part of the sternum and the pubic symphysis.
- Intravenous Injection directly into a superficial vein (Figs 11.2, 11.3).
- Intracardiac Injection directly into one of the chambers of the heart of an anaesthetised animal; the left ventricle is usually used.

COLLECTION OF SAMPLES

It is often necessary to analyse samples of blood,

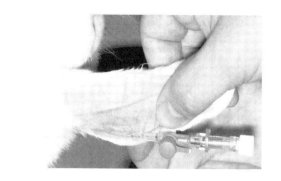

Fig. 11.3 Inserting butterfly needle into marginal ear vein.

urine or faeces in order to monitor reactions to experiments or to check health status.

Blood

Blood samples are often collected using the intravenous route although, for some experimental purposes, blood from an artery may be required. The method used depends on the species, the volume of blood required and whether it is to be sterile or not. Examples of methods are as follows.

Venesection

Collecting blood by cutting a superficial blood vessel is called venesection. When only a drop or two of blood is required from a mouse the animal may be placed in a restrainer with its tail protruding. The end of the tail should be cleaned with a skin disinfectant and treated with a surface acting local anaesthetic. A small nick is made in the end of the tail with a sterile scalpel blade or lancet. The drop of blood which forms on the tail can be transferred directly onto a slide for smearing or can be collected in a capillary tube. Pressure with a sterile swab can be applied to the wound to encourage clotting. If the technique is applied correctly the animal will suffer the minimum of discomfort.

Aspiration from a vein

If larger samples of sterile blood uncontaminated with tissue fluids are required, they are best obtained direct from the circulatory system by means of a hypodermic needle.

An adult rabbit may have several cm^3 of blood removed from an ear vein using the following technique. The rabbit is restrained by an assistant or placed into stocks. The ear should be shaved with clippers to make the vein more visible, and be disinfected to prevent infection. A surface acting local anaesthetic should be applied over the site. The vein may be dilated (raised) by warming or massaging the ear and occluding the vein close to the head with the finger and thumb.

A syringe fitted with a sterile needle of approximately 21 gauge and 1.5 inches in length is used to collect the sample. The skin is punctured and the vein entered so that the needle lies comfortably within the vein. As the vein is entered, blood may flow into the hub of the needle under venous pressure. Gentle aspiration using the syringe plunger will allow collection of the blood sample. Care must be taken not to apply too much suction as this could damage the blood cells and collapse the vein. When the collection is complete, pressure applied to the base of the ear should be removed and the needle withdrawn. Pressure should be applied with a sterile swab over the wound for a few seconds to allow the formation of a clot to prevent further blood loss.

Cardiac puncture

If relatively large samples of blood are required from species which have no readily accessible superficial veins, e.g. guinea pig or Syrian hamster, it can be obtained directly from the heart of an anaesthetised animal. Access to the heart is usually gained from the ventral surface by introducing the needle between the ribs directly above the ventricles.

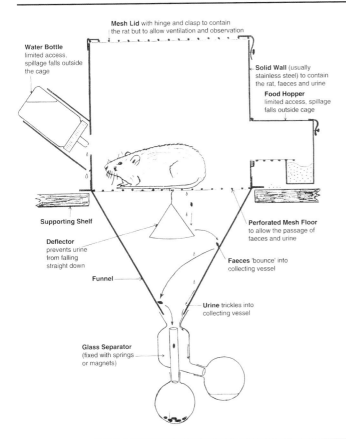

Mesh Lid with hinge and clasp to contain the rat but to allow ventilation and observation

Water Bottle
limited access, spillage falls outside the cage

Solid Wall (usually stainless steel) to contain the rat, faeces and urine

Food Hopper
limited access, spillage falls outside cage

Supporting Shelf

Perforated Mesh Floor
to allow the passage of faeces and urine

Deflector
prevents urine from falling straight down

Faeces 'bounce' into collecting vessel

Funnel

Urine trickles into collecting vessel

Glass Separator
(fixed with springs or magnets)

Fig. 11.4 Metabolism cage.

Faeces and urine, and measurement of food and water intake

Metabolism cages

The term 'metabolism cage' is used to describe specially designed or adapted cages which allow the collection of the urine and/or the faeces produced by an animal. However, strictly speaking the term 'metabolism cage' should be reserved for a cage system that allows much fuller measurement of more aspects of metabolism. A simple cage for the separate collection of faeces and urine from a rat is illustrated (Fig. 11.4, Plate 8). Such cages are generally only used for short term collections, e.g. overnight or for 24 hours.

These cages also allow accurate assessment of food and water consumption. However, the perfect feeders, waterers and separators have not yet been invented and some degree of mixture of food, water, faeces and urine does occur.

All metabolism apparatus needs to be kept scrupulously clean to avoid contamination of the samples. The samples of urine and faeces will deteriorate and should, therefore, be harvested at frequent intervals.

Chapter 12
Euthanasia

Euthanasia means quiet, easy death. It is the duty of animal technicians to make sure that, when the need arises, the animals in their charge are killed humanely. Whatever the reason for killing, operators must be proficient and confident in their ability to bring about a rapid and painless loss of consciousness followed by death.

Animals should never be killed in the presence of any other animals as the sounds, sights and odours produced during euthanasia will be stressful to them.

A laboratory animal may have to be killed because:

- It has come to the end of its economic breeding life.
- It is surplus to requirement, e.g. too old or too large.
- It has a severe injury.
- It or the colony it is in is affected by disease.
- It is in pain that cannot be alleviated.
- Its death is a requirement of a scientific project.

Many factors are involved in the choice of methods of euthanasia including:

- Species.
- Age.
- Size.
- Temperament and condition of the animal.
- Number of individuals to be killed.
- Availability of materials or apparatus.
- Reason for killing.
- Destiny of the carcass.
- Necessary urgency.

- Personal preferences, skills and strength of the operator.

LEGAL CONSIDERATIONS

In the UK euthanasia of animals used in scientific procedures is controlled by the Animals (Scientific Procedures) Act 1986. All methods of euthanasia are regulated procedures unless they are listed in Schedule 1 of the Act. Methods listed in Schedule 1 can be carried out by any competent person, except for the use of captive bolt guns and free bullets, which can only be used by licensed slaughtermen or veterinary surgeons competent in their use. The certificate holder of designated premises must ensure that a register of competent persons is kept. The register details the methods an individual is competent to perform and the species he/she is competent to use them on.

Any method of euthanasia not listed in Schedule 1 requires authorisation from the Home Office given in the form of a project and personal licence or as a special condition added to the certificate of designation. All workers who have to kill laboratory animals should ensure they are familiar with the details of the current Schedule 1.

METHODS OF EUTHANASIA

What follows is not intended to be used as an instruction manual. The intention of this section is to provide an understanding of the range of methods in use. Skill in performing euthanasia can only be gained by instruction from an experienced colleague.

All methods mentioned here are illustrated in the IAT video *Euthanasia with Care*. Methods in common use for killing laboratory animals are grouped into manual, other physical and chemical methods.

Manual methods

These may be distasteful to the operator but are often the quickest and appear to be least stressful for the animal. Such methods cannot be used if the brain and/or spinal cord are required for examination.

The high level of skills required to use these methods is gained by practice on surplus animals that have been killed by chemical means.

Dislocation of the neck

Mouse – An adult mouse may be killed by holding it by the base of the tail and allowing the front feet to grip a suitable surface such as a cage top or cork board. A rod, such as a strong ballpoint pen, is placed behind the ears and pressed down onto the neck whilst the hind end of the mouse is raised to about 30–40° from the horizontal and a firm pull exerted. During stretching, the dislocation can be felt through the hands of the operator.

Rat – A variation of the technique used for mice may be applied to post-weaner rats although older rats, particularly males, are too tough. Instead of a pen, a stronger instrument, e.g. a metal rod, is needed. It is often advisable to grip the hind legs as well as the tail.

Guinea pig – The guinea pig is placed on the bench and turned to face the operator. A hand is placed over its head and the first and second fingers are slid down the sides of the neck and are bent under the angles of the jaw. The guinea pig is lifted clear of the bench and the body is swung down rapidly, 'flicking' the wrist. The weight of the body dislocates the neck.

Rabbit – Weaned rabbits up to about 1 kg bodyweight may be killed by the so-called 'rabbit punch'. Older rabbits may be too large or too tough for this method. The rabbit is taken from the bench and suspended in one hand by the back legs. The other hand is used to deliver a 'karate chop' onto the base of the skull behind the ears. Some operators prefer to use a suitable heavy stick or other instrument instead of the hand.

Concussion (stunning) by striking the back of the head

Concussion causes unconsciousness quickly but does not necessarily cause death. Death must be assured by dislocation of the neck or bleeding out (exsanguination). Mice, rats and guinea pigs can be lifted by the base of the tail and/or hindquarters, turned over and the base of the skull struck onto a solid object such as the sharp edge of the bench.

Other physical methods

These include the captive bolt pistol, free bullet, electrocution and electrical stunning, which are normally not suitable for the species covered in this book.

With most physical methods of euthanasia there is involuntary movement of the animal after it is incapable of feeling any sensation. This may account for the operator dislike until he/she understands that the animal is not suffering any pain or distress.

Chemical methods

Inhalation

Inhalation methods may be unacceptable for some experimental work as lung tissues may be damaged and blood gas levels changed.

Euthanasia by inhalation is not normally recommended for animals of less than 10 days old or of a bodyweight of more than 1.5 kg. In young animals killing by this method takes a very long time; in large animals death also takes a long time and animals panic.

There is only one commonly used agent for

euthanasia by inhalation – carbon dioxide – although any animal that is undergoing an experimental procedure under inhalation anaesthesia may be killed by an overdose of the anaesthetic.

The gas carbon dioxide is one-and-a-half times heavier than air; it does not burn and will, in fact, extinguish flames; it has no smell and no colour. An animal exposed to carbon dioxide in a rising concentration will fairly quickly fall into a state of unconsciousness without excitation. The animals should be left in the carbon dioxide mixture for at least ten minutes and death must be confirmed by waiting until *rigor mortis* has set in, or death must be ensured by bleeding out or dislocating the neck before the disposal of the carcasses.

There are several means of administering carbon dioxide. Purpose-built chambers, which allow a regulated flow of carbon dioxide, are used. Such chambers allow a steady build-up of carbon dioxide without causing noise from the cylinder or a rapid change of temperature to distress the animals (Fig. 12.1). The chamber must be cleaned between each group of animals being killed and the chamber should be free from residual carbon

dioxide as immediate exposure to carbon dioxide produces panic in animals because of the sudden lack of oxygen.

A large plastic bag may also be used as a container for carbon dioxide by placing a cage holding the animal or a small group of animals within the bag. Most of the air should be removed and the bag slowly inflated with carbon dioxide. In this case, the bag should have a capacity of at least five times that of the cage or the carbon dioxide must be passed into the bottom of the cage and most of the air displaced.

The use of solid carbon dioxide (Cardice, Drikold) should not be used as a source of carbon dioxide for euthanasia as temperature and gas concentrations are not controllable.

Oral and parenteral administration

The chemical of choice is sodium pentobarbitone. Following administration, all the body tissues will contain the chemical which may preclude its use for some experiments.

Oral administration of Nembutal capsules – Uptake of the drug is slow and, although the animal does not become excited, it takes a considerable time for sleep, unconsciousness and death to occur. The principal value of this method is for dealing with intractable animals. When the unconscious state has been reached, it is advisable to accelerate the death of the animal by means of a parenteral injection of sodium pentobarbitone.

Parenteral administration – Sodium pentobarbitone (available as Euthatal, Lethobarb, Nembutal, Sagatal) may be given by either the intraperitoneal, intravenous or intracardiac route. Intraperitoneal injection is quicker than oral administration but the intravenous and intracardiac routes produce almost instantaneous unconsciousness and subsequent death.

Intravenous and intracardiac injection techniques are preferred for their speed of action but require considerable skill to perform. These injections must be given relatively quickly in order to overcome the excitation phase that occurs with such types of drug and it is important not to

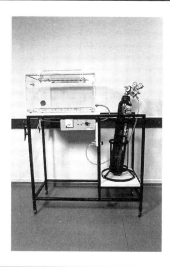

Fig. 12.1 A euthanasia cabinet for use with carbon dioxide.

inject into any other tissues as this causes extreme irritation.

RECOGNITION OF SIGNS OF DEATH

Signs that indicate an animal has died include lack of movement, lack of breathing, lack of reflexes, lack of heartbeat, lack of blood pressure, change of skin coloration to a blue tinge and involuntary urination or defaecation.

It is unsafe to assume that the presence of any of these indicators necessarily means that the animal has died. *Rigor mortis*, stiffening of the skeletal muscles, occurs after death and may be taken as conclusive evidence of death.

Before disposing of cadavers it is necessary to ensure death either by waiting for the onset of *rigor mortis* or by physical means such as exsanguination or cervical dislocation.

Chapter 13
The Animals (Scientific Procedures) Act 1986

It is a criminal offence to perform *regulated procedures* on *protected animals* unless they are done in accordance with the *Animals (Scientific Procedures) Act 1986* (the Act).

Those who wish to use animals for regulated procedures must demonstrate that there is no alternative for their work and that the benefits arising from their studies justify the use of animals. In addition, experiments must be designed so that animal suffering is minimised.

The Act is administered by the Secretary of State for the Home Office who enforces it through a system of certificates and licences. Establishments where animals are used, bred or supplied for regulated procedures must hold a *certificate of designation*. All programmes of work that include regulated procedures on protected animals must be covered by a *project licence* and all people who perform the regulated procedures on protected animals must hold a *personal licence*.

EXPLANATION OF TERMS

Protected animal

Not every animal is protected; the Act defines a protected animal as any living vertebrate (except man) and also includes the invertebrate *Octopus vulgaris*. Foetal, larval and embryonic forms of mammals, birds and reptiles are protected from halfway through their gestation or incubation periods. Amphibians, fish and *Octopus vulgaris* are protected from the point when they are capable of independent feeding.

Living

The Act states that an animal continues to live until its circulation has permanently ceased or its brain has been destroyed.

Regulated procedure

A regulated procedure is any experimental or other scientific procedure applied to a protected animal which may have the effect of causing that animal pain, suffering, distress or lasting harm.

A procedure is regulated even if the animal is rendered insensitive to pain and distress by the use of anaesthetic, sedative or by removal of part of the brain. In these cases the process of making the animal insensitive forms part of the regulated procedure.

Procedures which are not regulated

The Act specifically exempts some procedures from being regulated, including:

- Using a standard technique to identify animals (e.g. with rings, tags or tattoos) which is not a regulated procedure as long as it only causes momentary pain, does not cause lasting harm and the only purpose is to identify the animal.
- Recognised veterinary, agricultural or animal husbandry practices (e.g. castration, taking blood for diagnostic purposes and administration of medicines) are not regulated procedures provided they do not form part of a scientific study.

- Methods of euthanasia in designated premises which are listed in Schedule 1 of the Act.

DESIGNATED ESTABLISHMENTS

Three types of premises can be granted a certificate of designation under the Animals (Scientific Procedures) Act 1986: Designated Scientific Procedure Establishment, Designated Breeding Establishment and Designated Supplying Establishment.

Regulated procedures may only be performed in premises that have been designated, by the Secretary of State, as Scientific Procedure Establishments. The Secretary of State has the authority to vary this requirement if it is essential to the study; for instance, he may permit work to be carried out in a field or river.

Animals listed in Schedule 2 of the Act must be obtained from Designated Breeding or Supplying Establishments (although the Secretary of State has the power to authorise animals to be obtained from other sources). As the name suggests, designated breeding establishments breed animals specifically for use in regulated procedures. Designated suppliers obtain animals from various authorised sources and pass them on to designated scientific procedure establishments for use in regulated procedures. If scientific procedure establishments breed their own animals for use in regulated procedures they must also be designated breeders.

The Secretary of State has the power to vary animals listed in Schedule 2 of the Act, and has done so several times since it was first introduced. Animals in Schedule 2 fall into two groups; currently they are:

- Animals that must be obtained from designated breeders or suppliers – mice, rats, hamsters, gerbils, guinea pigs, rabbits, ferrets, primates, European quail, genetically modified sheep and pigs.
- Animals that must be obtained from designated breeders – cats and dogs.

Establishments wishing to become designated must satisfy the Secretary of State that their standards of accommodation and animal care meet those laid down in the current Codes of Practice for the Housing and Care of Animals used in Scientific Procedure Establishments or for the Housing and Care of Animals in Designated Breeding and Supplying Establishments (see Chapter 3). If the Secretary of State is satisfied with the standard of the establishment a certificate of designation is issued to an individual who represents the governing authority of the establishment. This person, named the Certificate Holder, is responsible for ensuring that the Act is correctly applied in the establishment and conditions attached to the certificate are observed.

The certificate holder's specific responsibilities include:

- Ensuring the fabric of the building is maintained in accordance with the Code of Practice.
- Providing the Home Office inspector with reasonable access to the establishment.
- Ensuring named persons carry out their duties effectively.
- Ensuring no unauthorised procedures take place in the establishment.
- Establishing a local ethical review procedure.
- Establishing a register of people competent to use Schedule 1 methods of euthanasia.
- Paying annual fees in connection with the Act.

The Act requires the certificate holder to nominate a named animal care and welfare officer (NACWO) and a named veterinary surgeon (NVS) (or in exceptional circumstances, other suitably qualified experts).

NACWOs are responsible to the certificate holder for the day-to-day care of animals in designated premises. They are expected to have expert knowledge and suitable experience of animal technology.

The current Home Office Guidance on the Animals (Scientific Procedures) Act 1986 states that named animal care and welfare officers should:

- Be familiar with the main provisions of the Act.
- Have an up-to-date knowledge of laboratory animal technology; be aware of the standards of

care, accommodation, husbandry and welfare set out in the relevant Codes of Practice; and take steps to ensure these are met.

- Be knowledgeable about relevant methods of humane killing listed in Schedule 1 of the Act (together with any other approved methods listed in the certificate of designation), and either be competent in their use or be able to contact others, named on a register maintained at the establishment, who are competent.
- Know which areas of the establishment are listed on the certificate of designation and the purposes for which their use is approved.
- Ensure that every protected animal kept in a designated holding area is seen and checked at least once a day by a competent person.
- Know how to contact, at any time, the named veterinary surgeon (or other suitable qualified person) or deputy and the certificate holder (or nominee). At designated scientific procedure establishments, the NACWO should also know how to contact project and personal licence holders.
- Be familiar with the main provisions of the project licences, particularly the adverse effects expected for each protocol, and the control measures and humane end points specified.
- Assist the certificate holder in ensuring that suitable records are maintained, under the supervision of the veterinary surgeon, of the health of protected animals; of the environmental conditions in the rooms in which protected animals are held; and of the source and disposal of protected animals.
- Take an active part in the ethical review process at the establishment, and advise applicants for licences and licensees on practical opportunities to implement the replacement, reduction and refinement alternatives.

The named veterinary surgeon is accountable to the certificate holder for the provision of expert advice on the health and welfare of protected animals. The specific responsibilities of the NVS include:

- Being familiar with the main provisions of the Act.

- Ensuring adequate veterinary cover is available at all times.
- Visiting all parts of the designated premises at a frequency that will allow the effective monitoring of the health status of animals.
- Being familiar with relevant methods of humane killing listed in Schedule 1 of the Act, together with any additional approved methods set out in the conditions of the certificate of designation.
- Having a thorough knowledge of the husbandry and welfare requirements of the species kept at the establishment (including the prevention, diagnosis and treatment of disease); and being able to advise on quarantine requirements and health screening, and the impact of housing and husbandry systems on the welfare needs of a protected animal.
- Controlling, supplying and directing the use of controlled drugs, prescription only medicines and other therapeutic substances for use on protected animals.
- Maintaining animal health records relating to all the protected animals at the establishment and ensuring that the records are readily available to the NACWO, the certificate holder and the Home Office.
- Certifying that an animal is fit to travel to a specified place.
- Having regular contact with the certificate holder and NACWO.
- Taking an active part in the ethical review process.
- Advising licensees on methods of anaesthesia, surgical technique and recognition of pain, suffering, distress or lasting harm.

Local ethical review procedure

All certificate holders have to establish a local ethical review process (LERP) in their establishments. The main purposes of the review are to provide the certificate holder and licensees with independent advice on animal welfare and ethical issues. A major part of the work of the procedure is concerned with examining project licence applications, the implementation of the principles of reduction, replacement and refinement and ensuring that staff are provided with relevant and up-to-date information on ethical and legal matters and best animal house practice.

The people included in the ethical review process include a named veterinary surgeon, named animal care and welfare officers, project and personal licensees and one or more 'lay persons'.

PROJECT LICENCES

A project licence authorises a programme of work that includes specified regulated procedures being performed on specified protected animals. Project licences will only be issued if the purpose of the work is for one or more of the following reasons:

- The prevention, diagnosis or treatment of disease.
- The study of physiology.
- Environmental protection benefiting health and welfare.
- Advancement of biological or behavioural sciences.
- Education and training.
- Forensic enquiries.
- Breeding animals for scientific purposes (if the resulting animals will express harmful mutations or the breeding involves genetic manipulations).

The person who will be responsible for the study must apply to the Home Office for a project licence. The application must state:

- The aims of the project and the potential benefits of the work.
- A description of the techniques that are to be used.
- The number and species of animals that are to be used (special justification must be given if cats, dogs or equines and primates are to be used).
- Justification for the use of animal models for the work.
- The degree of severity associated with each

procedure and the cumulative severity of the project.
- The designated premises where the project will be carried out.

Schedule 2A of the Act requires all experiments to be carried out under general or local anaesthesia unless applying the anaesthesia would be more traumatic than the experiment itself or if anaesthesia would be incompatible with the object of the experiment – in which case authorisation not to use anaesthetic must be given in the project licence.

Severity

Severity refers to the degree of pain, suffering, distress or lasting harm an animal experiences during the project. An assessment must be made of the maximum degree of severity any of the animals on the project may experience.

Severity is stated in one of four bands:

(1) *Unclassified* – animals are decerebrate or anaesthetised throughout the procedure and are not allowed to regain consciousness before they are killed.
(2) *Mild* – examples of which could be infrequent blood samples from a superficial vein and minor surgical procedures under anaesthesia.
(3) *Moderate* – examples include screening and development of potential pharmaceutical agents, most surgical procedures provided they are followed with suitable post-operative analgesia.
(4) *Substantial* – procedures which result in a major departure from the animal's usual state of health or well-being.

Benefit and severity

When deciding if a project licence should be granted, the Secretary of State weighs up the potential benefits of the research with the possible suffering of the animal. The degree of severity must always be the minimum consistent with the objectives of the study. The harmful effects on the animal can be minimised by appropriate use of analgesics and by introducing humane end points, that is withdrawing an animal from the study before it experiences harmful effects.

Project licence holder

If the Secretary of State is satisfied that the project is suitable he will grant a project licence which lasts for five years. The project licence applicant becomes the project licence holder. Attached to the licence are a set of conditions that are common to all projects, but any individual project may have extra conditions attached.

The project licence holder is responsible for the direction, management and supervision of the project. Specific responsibilities include:

- Ensuring the project is conducted legally and in accordance with the conditions of the project licence.
- Ensuring only authorised species and numbers of animals are used.
- Ensuring that personal licensees have the authority for the regulated procedures which they carry out as part of the project.
- Ensuring that personal licensees receive appropriate training, guidance and supervision.
- Ensuring that full and accurate records are kept.
- Submitting a statistical return to the Home Secretary of regulated procedures carried out for the project each year.

PERSONAL LICENCES

A personal licence authorises an individual to perform named regulated procedures on named protected animals at specified designated establishments. Regulated procedures listed on a personal licence can only be performed if they are also authorised by a project licence.

Personal licence applicants must fulfil the following criteria:

- Be at least 18 years of age.
- They must know how to perform the techniques

they are seeking permission to do on the species concerned.
- They must know the signs of pain, suffering or distress in those species.
- They should know how to care for the animals and the need for aftercare following a procedure.
- They must have appropriate education and training (the minimum education is normally the equivalent of five GCSEs at grade C or above; however, if a less well qualified person has the necessary skill to carry out a technique it is possible to issue a restricted licence).
- Potential licensees must attend an approved licensee training course.

People who satisfy these criteria are eligible to apply to the Secretary of State for a personal licence. A sponsor, who is able to confirm that the applicant fulfils the criteria above and that he/she is a suitable person to hold a licence, must sign the application form. The sponsor will normally be a senior member of the staff at the workplace of the applicant, who is also a project or personal licence holder.

When a personal licence is issued the personal licensee can perform his/her authorised procedures on any project that requires them; however it is usual to restrict new licensees to named projects for an initial period. Personal licences are reviewed every five years.

Conditions of personal licences

Standard conditions are attached to all personal licences and the Secretary of State may add any extra conditions that are appropriate. It is essential that all personal licensees are familiar with the conditions attached to their licences as failure to comply with some constitutes a criminal offence and could lead to the licence being revoked.

The responsibilities placed on personal licensees by the conditions include:

- Taking primary responsibility for the animals they have performed regulated procedures on.
- Ensuring the regulated procedures they per-

form are authorised by project and personal licences.

- Using appropriate sedatives, anaesthetics and analgesics to minimise pain, suffering and distress.
- Making arrangements for the care and welfare of animals during their absence.
- Making sure that where an animal is in severe pain or severe distress that cannot be alleviated it is painlessly killed by an appropriate method.
- Monitoring the degree of severity on the effects of procedures and informing the project licensee if permitted levels are, or could be, exceeded.
- Obtaining veterinary advice and treatment when necessary.
- Labelling cages and pens.
- Keeping records of animals and the procedures used on them and passing them to the project licensee so they can be incorporated into the annual returns to the Home Office.
- Adhering to the requirements of a supervisor if the personal licensee requires supervision.

NON-TECHNICAL PROCEDURES

Some aspects of regulated procedure are deemed to require no technical knowledge and present no risk of an animal suffering immediate pain, suffering, distress or lasting harm. Personal licensees may ask non-licensed assistants to perform these tasks, providing permission to do so has been granted on their personal licences. The Home Office gives illustrations of the type of work included in this definition and they are reproduced below. They do not include the normal feeding, watering, cleaning and other routine work of an animal unit, which does not require Home Office permission to complete.

Non-technical procedures which may be carried out by non-licensed assistants acting in accordance with precise and specific instructions from a suitably authorised personal licence holder who must remain within reach for assistance and advice if required are as follows:

(1) The filling of food hoppers and water bottles with previously mixed diets or liquids of altered constitution or to which test substances have been previously added.

(2) The placing of animals in some previously set-up altered environments, e.g. inhalation chambers, pressure chambers, aquatic environments.

(3) Pressing the exposure button to deliver previously determined doses of irradiation to an animal.

(4) Pairing/grouping associated with the breeding of animals with harmful genetic defects.

(5) Withdrawal of contents from an established ruminal fistula.

(6) Operating automated machinery which carries out inoculation of eggs.

(7) Placement of animals in restraining devices, as defined by the project licence.

(8) Withdrawal of food and/or water, as defined by the project licence.

(9) Placement of avian eggs into previously set chillers at the termination of a procedure.

The following tasks can only be undertaken by assistants in the presence of a suitably authorised personal licensee:

(10) In animals rendered insentient by decerebration or general anaesthesia, which is to persist until death, and through an established catheter, administration of a substance(s) as defined by the project licence or removal of body fluids.

(11) In animals rendered insentient by decerebration or general anaesthesia, which is to persist until death, the administration of electric stimuli through electrodes implanted by a personal licensee.

HOME OFFICE INSPECTORS

The Secretary of State has a team Home Office inspectors to help enforce the Act. They are either registered veterinary surgeons or registered medical practitioners. Certificate holders must allow them entry into designated premises at any reasonable time, but if there is reason to believe the Act is being breached a police constable with a magistrate's warrant may gain access at any time;

the constable must be accompanied by a Home Office inspector.

The duties of a Home Office inspector include:

• Advising the Secretary of State on applications for personal and project licences.
• Advising the Secretary of State on applications for certificates of designation.
• Visiting designated premises to ensure the law is being complied with.
• Reporting any deviation from the law or conditions attached to certificates or licences to the Secretary of State and recommending suitable action to be taken.

If it appears to an inspector that the effects of a procedure on an animal are too severe or that the animal is suffering considerable pain or distress, the inspector can direct that the animal is removed from the procedure and given suitable treatment or painlessly killed. It is an offence not to comply with this instruction by the inspector.

ANIMAL PROCEDURES COMMITTEE (APC)

The APC is appointed by the Secretary of State to advise him on matters covered by the Act. The committee produces an annual report which the Secretary of State presents to Parliament. The APC is made up of an assortment of people, both licensees and non-licensees, appointed according to a procedure laid down in the Act.

HOME OFFICE PUBLICATIONS

The Secretary of State orders publication of documents concerned with the operation of the Animals (Scientific Procedures) Act 1986:

(1) Guidance on the Operation of the Animals (Scientific Procedures) Act 1986 (HMSO 1999). This publication contains a full copy of the Act and provides more detailed guidance on its implementation.
(2) Code of Practice for the Housing and Care of Animals used in Scientific Procedures (HMSO 1989) and the Code of Practice for the Housing and Care of Animals in Designated Breeding and Supplying Establishments (HMSO 1995). These Codes set the standards of husbandry and care that are required under the Act.
(3) Code of Practice for the Humane Killing of Animals under Schedule 1 to the Animals (Scientific Procedures) Act 1986 (HMSO 1997). This code explains and comments on terms used in Schedule 1 of the Act.

In addition to these publications the Secretary of State publishes a statistical analysis of all procedures performed each year, based on the annual returns provided by project licensees and a report prepared by the Animal Procedures Committee.

Further information can be obtained from the Home Office website: http://www.homeoffice. gov.uk/ccpd/aps.htm.

Chapter 14
Handling and Sexing

Animal technicians must be able to handle, sex and restrain the animals in their care without alarming or harming them and without putting themselves at risk of injury. This chapter describes methods of handling and sexing that are in common use, but the level of skill expected of animal technicians cannot be gained by reading alone. Competence in animal handling can only be achieved by practice, under the supervision of a more experienced colleague.

The methods described in this chapter are demonstrated in the IAT video *Handle with Care*.

It is common to require handlers to wear protective clothing including gloves, masks and hats when handling laboratory animals. This limits exposure to laboratory animal allergens and reduces the risk of pathogens being transferred between animals and handlers.

GENERAL PRINCIPLES OF ANIMAL HANDLING

Animals should be approached in a confident and relaxed manner. They are usually calmed by being spoken to in a gentle voice. They must be held firmly so that they feel secure; animals that feel insecure become frightened, struggle and may become aggressive. The same reaction may result if they are held too tightly.

Animals that are handled well soon get used to it and often seek human contact. Where temporary close restraint is required it can be achieved by gently controlling the animal's head. Complex procedures are made less worrying for the animal if it undergoes a period of preparatory training.

Extra support is required for old, sick or pregnant animals.

As much care should be taken when putting animals back into their cages as when they are removed because it is possible for injuries to occur if they knock themselves on the edges or top of the door or lid as they go back into the cage.

There is no one correct way to handle an animal. The method used depends on four main variables: the animal, the design of cage or pen, the handler and the procedure being undertaken.

Animal	Techniques vary from species to species and with size, weight, age, temperament, condition of the animal and its location within the cage or pen.
Cage or pen	The design of cages and pens varies greatly; for instance, the cage may have a door or a removable lid, the cage floor may be solid or gridded, the depth of the cage may be shallow or large. All affect the way in which an animal can be removed from and returned to the cage.
Handler	People may be large or small, strong or weak, right-handed or left-handed, experienced or less experienced, all of which will affect the handling technique they choose to use.
Procedure to be undertaken	Animals are handled for a variety of reasons and techniques will differ if the animal is to be

removed to a clean cage, to be sexed or for a more complex procedure.

General principles of sexing

In young animals where the external sex organs are not obviously different, the ano-genital distances are often the main criteria for determining the sex of an individual. There is a longer distance between the anus and penis of the male than between the anus and genital opening of the female.

TECHNIQUES FOR INDIVIDUAL SPECIES

The animals covered in this chapter are mice, rats, Syrian hamsters, guinea pigs, rabbits, ferrets, cats and dogs.

The mouse

Handling

Adults: Individual animals may be picked up by the base of the tail but the weight of the animal should be supported on the hand or other surface as soon as possible. If any part of the tail other than the base is held, the mouse will be able to climb up and bite (Plate 9). Mice that are pregnant should be scooped up bodily, without squeezing, using both hands. Groups of mice may be transferred from one cage to another by scooping them up with both hands (Plate 10).

A mouse may be restrained by picking it up by the tail, and allowing it to grip a rough surface so it will pull away. The scruff of the neck may then be grasped with the thumb and fingers (Plate 11) and the hand turned so that the mouse lays on its back. The tail can be restrained with the little finger.

Very young mice: New-born mice are gently picked up bodily and several may be scooped up at a time.

Weanlings: As soon as young mice become very active, when they are about three weeks old, they may need to be held by the base of the tail in order to control them.

Sexing

Very young mice: the pups are held so that the genitalia can be inspected and the ano-genital distance and genital papillae can be compared. When body hair begins to grow the region surrounding the teats in the female remains hairless until approximately 16 days of age. This can help to identify females (Plates 12–17).

Weanlings: Ano-genital distances and the sizes of the genital papillae are used to distinguish between the sexes until about six weeks of age when the testes descend in the male. From then on males and females are easily distinguished.

The rat

Handling

Adults: Adult rats are picked up by placing the thumb and forefinger around their neck with the palm across the shoulders; the remaining fingers are placed around the chest to assist when lifting the animal (Plate 18). Larger rats must be supported by placing the other hand under the body when lifting. Adult rats can be restrained by gently increasing the finger and thumb pressure around the neck and using the thumb to control the jaw (Plate 19). An alternative method of restraint is to adopt a method of scruffing similar to that described for a mouse. The hind legs and/or tail must be supported and restrained by the other hand. Small groups of young rats can be transferred from one cage to another by scooping them up with both hands.

Very young rats: Rat pups should be handled in the way described for mice of a similar age but, by the time they are two weeks old, the best method is to pick them up bodily as, at this stage, the tails are particularly delicate.

Sexing

Rats are sexed in the same way as mice but as the animals are larger the ano-genital distance and genital papillae are also proportionally larger (Plates 20–27).

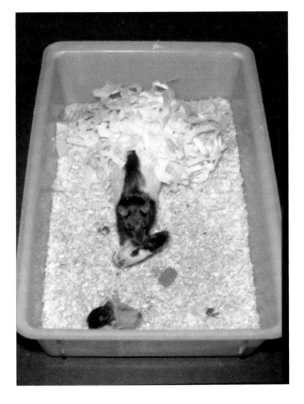

Plate 1 Female rat retrieving pup.

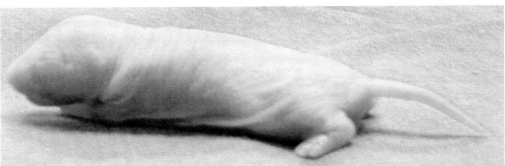

Plate 2 One day old rat. Eyes closed, pinna close to the head, no hair on body.

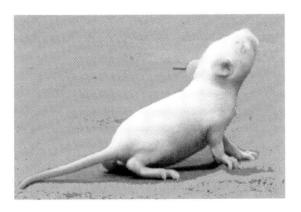

Plate 3 11 day rat. Eyes closed, pinna separating from head, body covered with short hair.

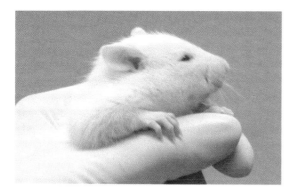

Plate 4 19 day old rat. Fully furred, ears separate from head.

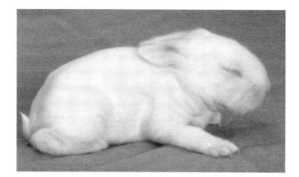

Plate 5 11 day old rabbit.

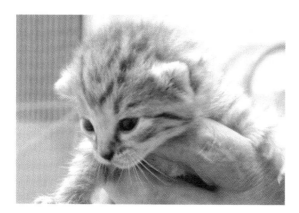

Plate 6 25 day old kitten–eyes open but ears still not fully separated.

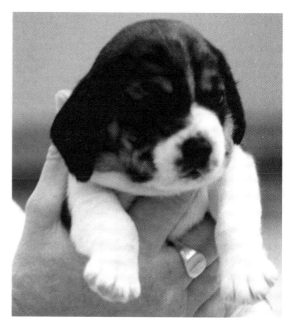

Plate 7 25 day old Beagle puppy.

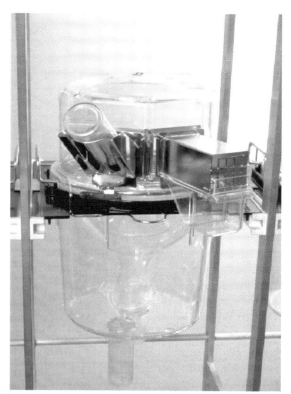

Plate 8 Metabolism cage.

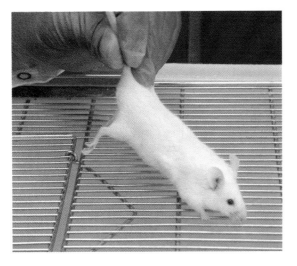

Plate 9 Picking up mouse by base of tail.

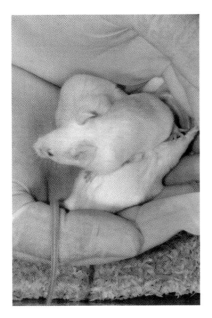

Plate 10 Moving mice by cupping in the hand.

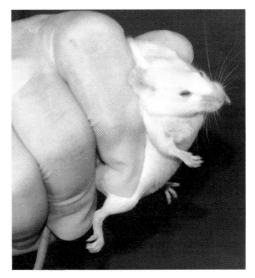

Plate 11 Scruffing mouse.

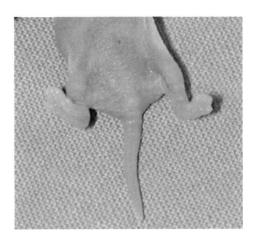

Plate 12 Day old female mouse.

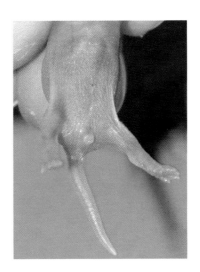

Plate 13 Day old male mouse.

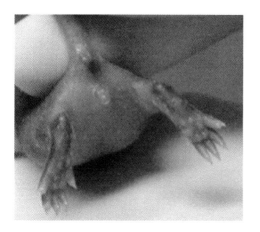

Plate 14 Male mouse, 10 days old.

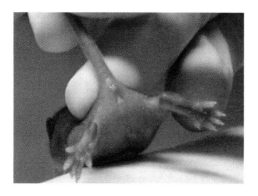

Plate 15 Female mouse, 10 days old.

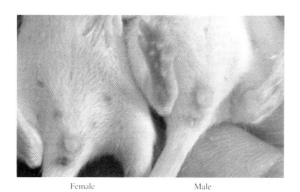

Female   Male

Plate 16 Weaner mice.

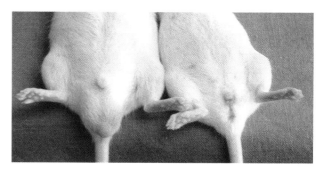

Plate 17 Adult male and female mice.

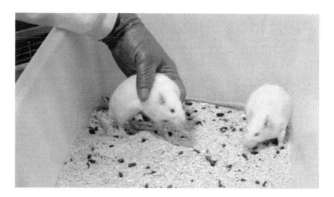

Plate 18 Picking up rat.

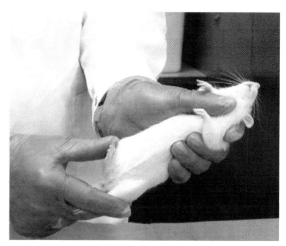

Plate 19 Restraining rat.

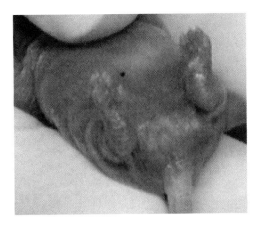

Plate 20 Female rat 1–2 days old.

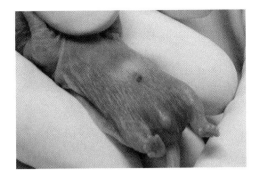

Plate 21 Male rat 1–2 days old–milk can be clearly seen in the stomach.

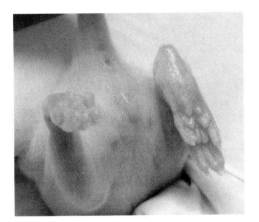

Plate 22 Female rat 10 days old.

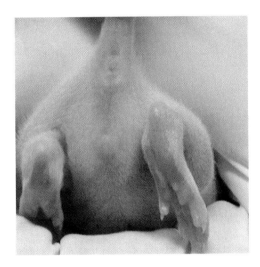

Plate 23 Male rat 10 days old.

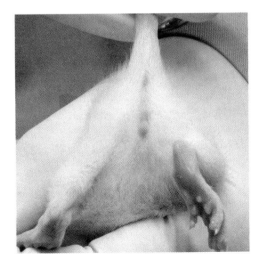

Plate 24 Female rat 19 days.

Plate 25 (*right*) Male rat 19 days.

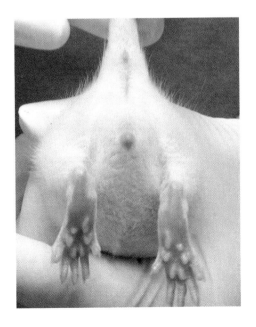

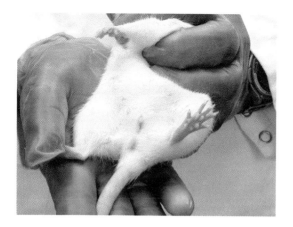

Plate 26 Adult female rat.

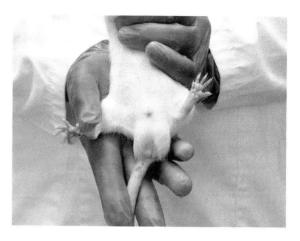

Plate 27 Adult male rat.

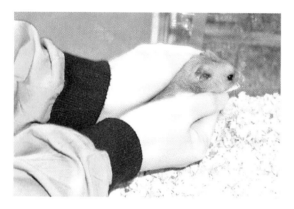

Plate 28 Cupping hamster.

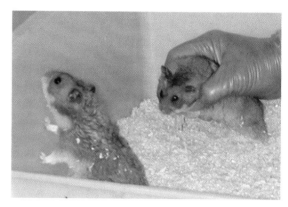

Plate 29 Taking hamster rom cage.

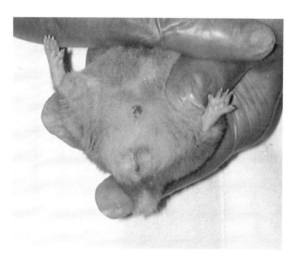

Plate 30 Male hamster.

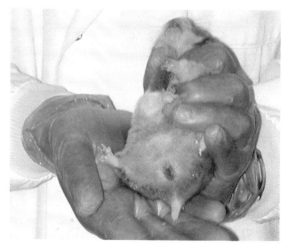

Plate 31 Female hamster.

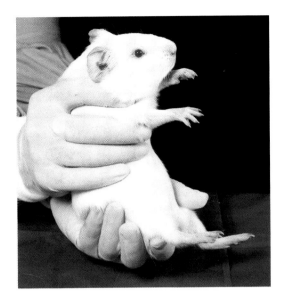

Plate 32 Holding a guinea pig.

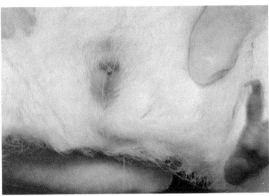

Plate 33 Adult female guinea pig.

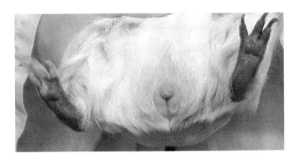

Plate 34 Adult male guinea pig.

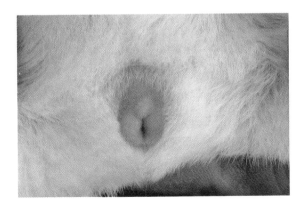

Plate 35 Immature male guinea pig.

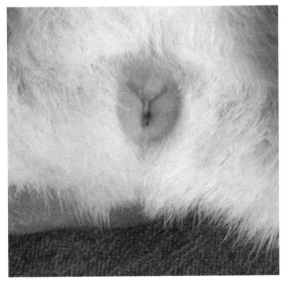

Plate 36 Immature female guinea pig.

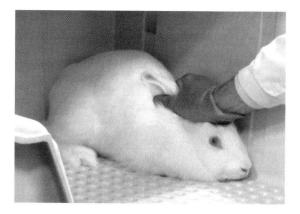

Plate 37 Taking rabbit from cage (1).

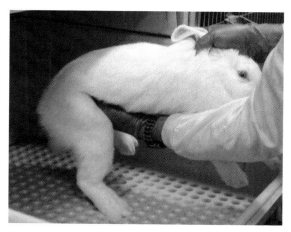

Plate 38 Taking rabbit from cage (2).

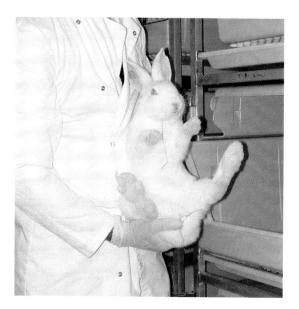

Plate 39 Holding rabbit for sexing.

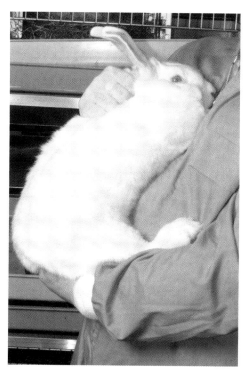

Plate 40 Carrying rabbit.

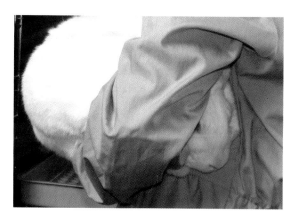

Plate 41 Rabbit in carrying position.

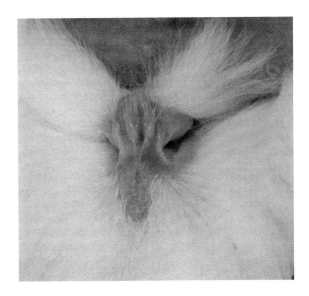

Plate 42 Immature female rabbit.

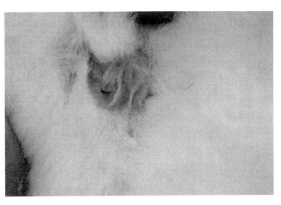

Plate 43 Immature male rabbit.

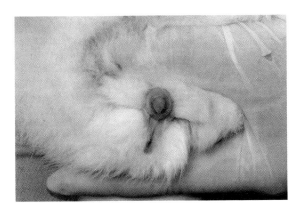

Plate 44 Adult male rabbit.

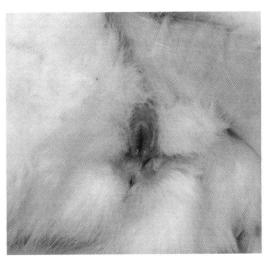

Plate 45 Adult female rabbit.

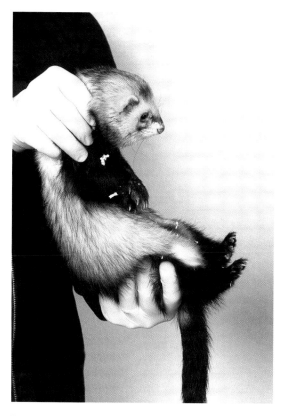

Plate 46 Holding ferret.

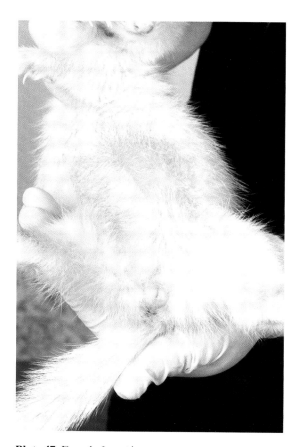

Plate 47 Female ferret in season.

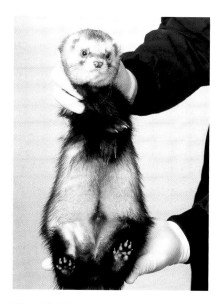

Plate 48 Male ferret.

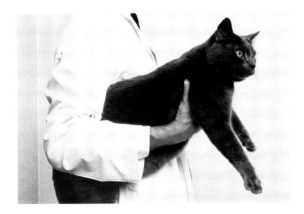

Plate 49 Carrying cat.

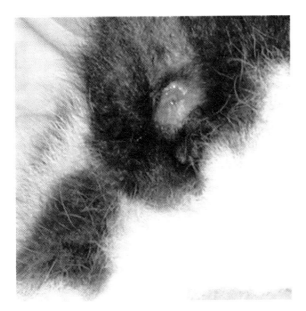

Plate 50 Female kitten.

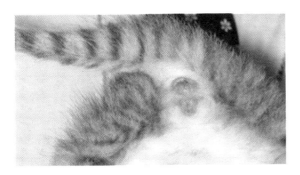

Plate 51 Male kitten.

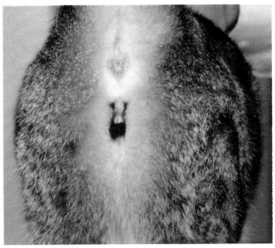

Plate 52 Adult female cat.

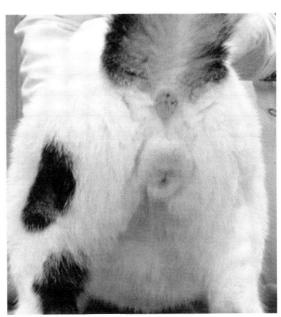

Plate 53 Adult male cat.

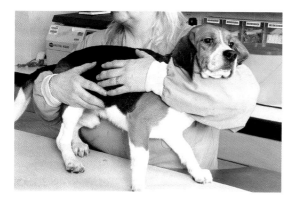

Plate 54 Lifting male dog from table.

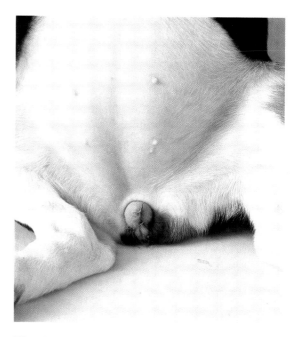

Plate 56 Female puppy.

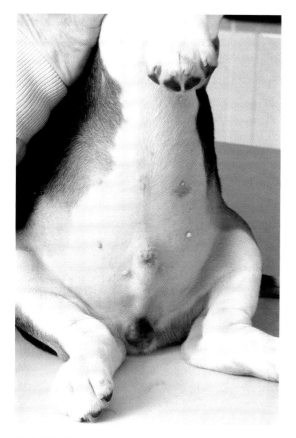

Plate 55 Male puppy.

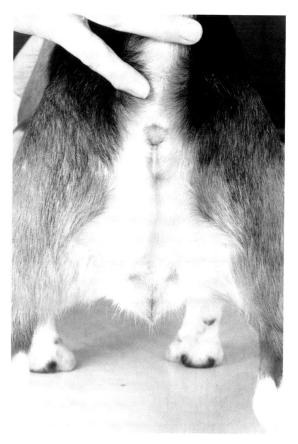

Plate 57 Adult bitch.

The Syrian hamster

Hamsters are nocturnal and are much more likely than mice and rats to be found asleep during the daytime. When disturbed in these circumstances they may roll onto their backs and give voice to their disapproval. They should be allowed to wake up fully before any attempt is made to pick them up.

Handling

Hamsters may be scooped up with one or both hands (Plates 28, 29) or may be picked up by the scruff. If it is necessary to restrain the animal a hind leg can be held between the fingers instead of the tail, a technique that is less straightforward and requires more practice than that used for mice.

Sexing

Adults: A hamster can be sexed whilst it is cupped in the hand by rolling it onto its back and turning the top hand so that the genital region is exposed. When adult male hamsters are upturned the testes and scrotal sacs are often not as obvious as in mice and rats but are obvious when the animal is moving in the cage. An initial impression of the sex of adults may be obtained from observing the shape of the rear end of the body when the animal is in the cage (Plates 30, 31).

Young and immature hamsters are sexed in the way described for mice of the same age.

The guinea pig

Guinea pigs are easily excited and become difficult to catch and handle if they are disturbed, so it is particularly important to approach them quietly.

Handling

Guinea pigs are picked up in the same way as the rat. The thumb and forefinger are placed around the neck with the palm of the hand across the shoulders; the remaining fingers are used to assist when lifting the animal (Plate 32). Larger guinea pigs should be supported at the rear end with the other hand. Extreme care should be taken when handling late-term pregnant guinea pigs. They may be lifted up after sliding one hand under the body between the forelegs and the other hand under the body between the hindlegs.

Sexing

The shape of the genital area of guinea pigs varies with the sexes (Plates 33–36). If gentle pressure is applied in front of the genital region of the male, the penis will be expressed but this is not necessary in order to tell the sexes apart. The teats are no guide to the sex of a guinea pig as those of the male are also fairly well developed.

The rabbit

Handling

The hind limbs of a rabbit are very powerful and, if the rabbit is allowed to kick, it may damage its spine or scratch the handler.

A rabbit can be safely removed from its cage by ensuring it is facing the handler, who can then pass a hand over the head to grasp the skin at the scruff of the neck. Keeping the ears in the hand can control the head (Plate 37). A second hand can control the hind limbs either by placing it behind the animal so it can be bunched up or by sliding the hand under the rabbit so that, as it is lifted, the back is straightened and the hind limbs extended slightly (Plate 38).

If the rabbit is to be carried any distance, it can be transferred to the chest of the handler without releasing the scruff and the second hand placed under the hindquarters to support the weight of the body (Plates 39, 40). Alternatively, the head can be tucked under the arm and the body well supported (Plate 41).

When returning a rabbit to its cage it is essential to prevent it from kicking with its hind limbs and this is done by returning it rear end first.

Sexing

An immature rabbit can be sexed by picking it up by its scruff while supporting its body by the second hand. The second hand can also be used to hold the tail back, and the thumb used to clear the fur around the genitalia (Plates 42, 43). Slight pressure applied to the genital region will expose the rudimentary penis with its round opening in the case of the male or the vaginal opening as a slit in the female. Mature rabbits may need to be supported on a table or the thigh of the handler. The sex difference is clear: in the female the vaginal opening and vulva are more obvious and, in the male, the penis and testicles will be clearly seen (Plates 44, 45).

In larger breeds and older animals, secondary sexual characteristics may be apparent: the female may have a dewlap and the male is generally thicker set with a 'squarer' head.

The ferret

Handling

Ferrets are very inquisitive and will come to the opened doors of their cages and extend their necks in order to see out. It is useful to distract the ferret with one hand whilst the other hand is used to grasp its neck using the thumb to control the lower jaw as if it were a rat. The hindquarters should be supported on lifting (Plate 46). The ferret has a long back which should be kept straight and often the forearm is used to support the body.

If the ferret is being approached from above it may be necessary to gently restrain the animal by the tail before grasping it by the neck.

Sexing

To the inexperienced, the swollen vulva of the female in oestrus may be mistaken for a scrotum. The position of the genitalia is similar to that of the dog and cat (Plates 47, 48). The bodyweight of adult ferrets varies considerably through the seasons.

The cat

Handling

Many people are frightened of the sharp claws and teeth of cats but laboratory cats are sufficiently tame for them to be picked up bodily in a similar way to that used for a pet cat (Plate 49). The scruff of the neck may be used as a means of gentle restraint or to control them if they have to be carried any distance. A similar technique to that used for a rabbit may be employed to remove a cat from the back of a cage.

Sexing

The size and shape of head and body can be used as a guide to sexing mature cats; the males tend to be larger and 'squarer'. Inspection of the genital region will reveal a clear difference between the sexes in both kittens and adults (Plates 50–53).

The dog

Handling

Breeds of dog vary considerably in size, and techniques for handling, therefore, need adaptation. The beagle, a medium-sized and commonly used dog, is illustrated. The confidence of the dog should initially be gained by eye contact and talking to it. Squatting down to approach the dog from its level can help to keep it calm. It can then be picked up bodily (Plate 54). As with the cat, the scruff may be used to control or restrain the dog.

Sexing

Inspection of the genital region will reveal a clear difference between the sexes in both puppies and adults. The penis and scrotal sac are usually obvious without picking the dog up (Plates 55–57).

Chapter 15
Safety

Laboratory animal facilities present many risks to the health and safety of people working within them and, in some cases, to people outside. This chapter is designed to provide a basic understanding and increased awareness of the risks and to indicate how they can be minimised. It is the responsibility of all employees to be aware of their employer's safety policy and practices and to co-operate in carrying them out.

THE HEALTH AND SAFETY AT WORK ACT 1974

The provision of a safe working environment is a legal requirement. The Health and Safety at Work Act 1974 puts a duty on employers to ensure, as far as reasonably practicable, the health, safety and welfare of employees while at work and to protect the health and safety of others from the activities carried out in the workplace. Employers must see that the work environment and work practices are safe and must also ensure that the employees are provided with information and training so that they are able to work safely.

Employees also have duties imposed on them by the Act. They must take reasonable care of their own health and safety and the health and safety of others who may be affected by their actions or omissions. They must co-operate with their employers to enable the employer to carry out their statutory duties. It is a criminal offence for an employee to misuse anything provided in the interests of health and safety.

A number of regulations have been issued under the Health and Safety at Work Act which detail the specific measures employers must take to ensure the health and safety of their employees. An important example of these is the Control of Substances Hazardous to Health Regulations.

Control of Substances Hazardous to Health Regulations 1999 (COSHH)

The COSHH regulations were introduced to prevent employees contracting work related disease resulting from the exposure to materials found to be hazardous. The regulations require employers to perform an adequate assessment of the risk to health and safety arising from a work activity associated with hazardous substances.

The term 'hazard' refers to the potential of a substance to cause harm. 'Risk' refers to the likelihood that a substance will harm given the circumstances of its use. A substance in this context is any material compound or mixture used or produced within the working environment. These include animal allergens, chemicals and dust from wood, flour, grain and hay.

Once the risks are established, control measures must be introduced and maintained so that they are reduced. Information, instruction and training must be given to all people affected to ensure that the control measures introduced are fully understood and complied with. The effectiveness of the control measures must be monitored on a regular basis and alterations introduced where necessary.

Under the COSHH regulations there is a requirement to monitor the health of employees if they are exposed to a substance that is associated with a particular disease or has adverse effects. All animal technicians are exposed on a daily basis to animal allergens, which in certain cases may develop into occupational asthma, and therefore they must undergo a regular programme of health surveillance.

PERSONAL CODE OF SAFETY IN THE ANIMAL UNIT

The principles underlying safe behaviour in the animal unit are based on all employees adopting a mature and responsible attitude. Standard work procedures put in place by employers must be adhered to and instructions followed conscientiously. Specified safety precautions should always be taken, e.g. wearing of protective clothing, and all staff must make themselves aware of emergency procedures in the event of an incident. Potentially hazardous tasks should only be tackled by suitably trained staff working with at least one other person.

Although tempting, playing practical jokes or 'larking around' with work colleagues are forbidden as these activities often have unfortunate consequences.

Personal hygiene

A high standard of personal hygiene must be maintained in an animal facility to prevent transmission of disease and accidental absorption or ingestion of harmful substances.

Storing food and drink in animal units, other than in separate designated areas, could result in them becoming contaminated with pathogens and other harmful substances. Eating and drinking in the unit could result in these substances becoming ingested. Smoking can also lead to ingestion of harmful substances and, in addition, is a fire hazard. Wearing and applying cosmetics makes the skin sticky and allows pathogens, chemicals and allergens to stick to it and remain in contact for a longer time.

To reduce the risk of contamination, hands must be washed after handling animals and animal products, even if gloves have been worn. Hands and faces should be washed and outer protective

clothing removed before entering designated eating and drinking areas in a facility.

Personal hygiene extends to the work area; worktops and other surfaces should be kept clean and be treated with a suitable disinfectant as soon as work has been completed.

Safe work practice

Working with live animals, chemicals or laboratory equipment carries risks. If things go wrong whilst someone is working alone these risks are made more serious because there is no one available to give, or to get, help. The higher the risks involved in any procedure, the more important it is not to work alone.

Machinery can be hazardous and must not be operated without prior training. Appropriate protective clothing, e.g. ear defenders (Fig. 15.1), respiratory protection and safety footwear, must be worn in order to minimise risks. Long hair and loose clothing, such as ties, may get caught in machinery with moving parts and cause severe injury. Safety guards fitted to machinery must not be removed even if it appears to make the job quicker or easier.

Whenever a task is being performed it is important to be aware of the possible hazards associated

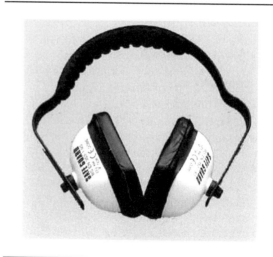

Fig. 15.1 Ear protectors.

with it. For example, using water to clean an area is effective but could be hazardous. Water produces aerosols and makes surfaces slippery especially if detergents or disinfectants are added. There is an additional hazard if electrical equipment is in the area. The risk can be controlled by:

- Removing electrical apparatus from the area before cleaning.
- Wearing appropriate non-slip footwear.
- Displaying warning signs in the immediate environment.
- Cleaning up excess water immediately and making the floor as dry as possible by using a squeegee or other suitable equipment.
- Reporting large spillages of water to a senior person.

Safe practice on leaving a work area, at the end of the working day or at break times, should ensure that:

- All animals are secure and have access to food and water.
- All naked flames are extinguished, ensuring that all Bunsen burners are disconnected from the gas taps.
- All non-essential electrical equipment is switched off.
- The area is left clean and tidy.
- All non-essential lighting is switched off.
- All doors are closed.

Manual handling

More than a quarter of all work accidents reported each year are associated with manual handling. Approximately 80% of the working population will suffer a back injury resulting in time taken off work; the majority of injuries result in more than three days absence. The most common forms of injury are strains and sprains to the lower back and arise over a period of time, not as a result of a single handling incident. Other injuries associated with manual handling include cuts, bruises, fractures and even amputations.

Employers have a responsibility to give training

to those required to lift objects. This training helps the individual to identify slip and trip hazards, assess the weight of loads to be lifted, use the correct lifting technique and identify the dangers of careless or unskilled methods of handling.

Injury can be avoided if the following control measures are implemented:

- Minimise manual handling where possible.
- Try to redesign the task to avoid moving the load or by using mechanical/electrical lifting equipment, e.g. pallet truck (if authorised to use them).
- If handling is unavoidable make a suitable assessment of the manual handling operation, including the load involved, how far it has to be moved, the immediate environment and then introduce sufficient safety measures.

Before commencing manual lifting and moving:

- Wear appropriate personal protective equipment (especially for the hands and feet).
- Be aware of personal limitations such as strength, age and fitness levels.
- Ensure that there is a clear route of passage without any obstructions.
- Consider any variations in levels of floors or work surfaces.
- Ensure adequate lighting along the route is provided.

When lifting, the following guidance should be followed:

- Hands should be kept clear from potential hazards and not placed on the outer edge of the load where they could be crushed.
- The load should be evenly distributed.
- The load should be gripped with the palm of the hand, not with the fingertips.
- Grip should not be changed during transportation.
- The weight should be held close to the body.
- Lift with the legs by bending the knees whilst maintaining a straight back.

- Keep the chin tucked in.
- Lift in easy stages, floor to knees, knees to carrying position.
- Reverse this process when setting the load down.
- Avoid twisting the back and maintain a clear vision over the top of the load.
- Where possible place the load onto a bench or table allowing room for the safe removal of the fingers.

Repetitive strain injuries

Prolonged repetition of a particular manual task, especially if it requires using force or holding the body in an awkward position, may lead to repetitive strain injuries (RSIs). Common signs are numbness, tenderness, pain, or pale cold skin in the affected area. Such injuries can be avoided by limiting repetitious tasks as much as possible, alternating hands, reducing the amount of force used or by paying attention to body position. It is important to take regular breaks, to move position, stretch and allow time for the body to recover.

INTERNATIONAL HAZARD WARNING SIGNS

Signs play an important part in warning people of the hazards associated with a process, substance or work area. The signs in use must conform to EU safety standards. Figures 15.2 and 15.3 illustrate some of these signs.

 EMERGENCY

 FIRE FIGHTING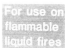

 PROHIBITION

 WARNING

Fig. 15.2 Examples of warning signs.

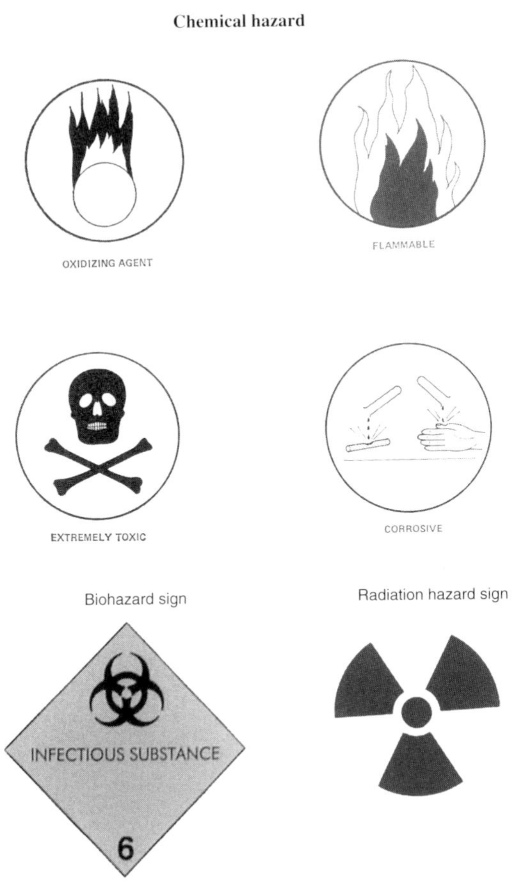

Chemical hazard

OXIDIZING AGENT

FLAMMABLE

EXTREMELY TOXIC

CORROSIVE

Biohazard sign

Radiation hazard sign

INFECTIOUS SUBSTANCE

6

Fig. 15.3 Examples of hazard signs.

- *Mandatory signs* (those that have to be obeyed) are blue and white, e.g. 'hearing protection must be worn'.
- *First aid and safety procedure signs* are green and white, e.g. first aid box, eye wash point, fire exit signs.
- *Prohibition signs* have a red circle with a red diagonal line, e.g. no smoking, mobile phones prohibited.
- *Fire fighting signs* are red, e.g. fire extinguisher, fire alarm point.
- *Warning signs* are yellow, e.g. caution high voltage, caution trip hazard.
- *Chemical warning signs* can be found on chemical containers.

LABORATORY ANIMAL ALLERGY

An allergen is a substance that stimulates a specific type of immune response in an individual. Common allergens are produced by arthropods (dust mites and insect bites), pollen and some foods. The hair, feathers, dander and urine of laboratory animals, particularly rats and mice, cause an allergic response in approximately 25% of people working with them.

The symptoms are often mild but can develop into potentially life threatening diseases like asthma. The severity of an allergic reaction increases with the frequency of the exposure and with the amount of allergen present.

Symptoms of allergy

These include:

- Eyes   Itchy, watery, red colour, swollen eyelids.
- Nose   Itchy, running, sneezing.
- Skin   Itching, cracked skin, blisters, nettle rash.
- Lungs   Coughing, wheezing, tightness of the chest, shortness of breath.

Because laboratory animal allergy is potentially very dangerous, people working with laboratory animals are required to undergo regular health checks so that signs can be picked up early. If any of the symptoms mentioned above are noticed they should be reported to a supervisor or to the Occupational Health Department so that the problem can be identified and action can be taken to avoid recurrence.

Measures can be taken to reduce exposure to allergens, including:

- Wearing face masks or ventilated air-flow helmets (Fig. 15.4).
- Good ventilation systems.
- Housing animals behind barriers such as individually ventilated cages or isolators.
- Regular cleaning of animal cages (in a cage cleaning station) and pens to prevent build up of allergens.

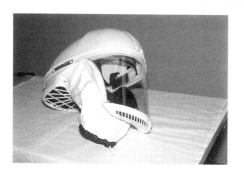

Fig. 15.4 Air flow helmet.

• Movement of animals within filtered containers.

Animal allergens can settle onto work clothes; to prevent contamination of people who do not normally come into direct contact with laboratory animals, personal protective clothing must be removed before leaving the facility or entering staff rest areas.

FIRE

Fire begins when three elements come together:

• Oxygen (usually in air but it can be supplied by oxidising chemicals).
• Sufficient heat to provide ignition.
• A fuel.

If one of these elements is absent there will be no fire. Methods of extinguishing fires work by removing one of the three elements, usually reducing heat or excluding oxygen.

Fires are divided into categories based on the fuel present and the way in which the fire can be extinguished:

Class A fires	Carbonaceous material that forms glowing embers, e.g. paper, wood, coal, cloth, plastics.
Class B1 fires	Liquids soluble in water, e.g. alcohol, acetone.
Class B2 fires	Liquids that are insoluble in water, e.g. petrol, oil, fats.
Class C fires	Gases and liquefied gases, e.g. butane, propane, methane.
Class D fires	Metals, e.g. magnesium, aluminium, sodium, potassium.
Class E fires	Fire involving electrical equipment.

Table 15.1 shows a range of fire extinguishers and the type of fire they are appropriate for. It is essential to select the appropriate extinguisher as using the wrong one can increase the danger to the individual and may make the situation worse. Since 1997 all new extinguishers are coloured red. The labels on these extinguishers must be checked to ensure the correct one is being used. Some older extinguishers may still be in use so the table includes the old colours.

Not only must the correct extinguishers be used, they must be used in the correct way so all staff should undergo fire fighting training. Staff should always follow instructions of local fire

Table 15.1 Fire extinguishers (type and colour of label) with type of fire for their use.

Type of fire (see text)	Foam Cream	ABC Powder Blue	Carbon dioxide Black	Water Red
A	Yes	Yes	Yes	Yes
B	Yes	Yes	Yes	No
C	No	Yes	Yes	No
D		Special dry powder		
E	No	Yes	Yes	No

officers on the most appropriate way to react to a fire.

Any door will stop smoke and even hold back the fire for a while. Closed doors restrict the supply of air which reduces the intensity of the fire. Doors designated as fire doors are specifically designed to retard the progress of a fire and therefore must be kept closed when not in use. Some fire doors include a strip of material that expands when heated to seal the gap around the door. Some are kept open by magnetic catches that are automatically released once the alarm is raised.

It is essential to know the positions of fire alarm buttons in any work area so that they may be used quickly in an emergency. The traditional alarm bell may not be used in animal units, particularly those containing small rodents, as the noise of a clanging bell distresses the animals. Instead some units are fitted with flashing light warning systems in every room or with 'Silentone' devices that give a 'Dee-dar' or warbling sound which does not upset the animals. Some alarm systems give a ring with intermittent sounds or lights, designed to prepare people to evacuate, and a continuous warning which means 'go now'.

Staff must familiarise themselves with the nearest fire exit and the designated assembly points outside the building. Fire exits must be kept free from obstruction and be properly signed.

If a fire is discovered it is imperative that the alarm is raised immediately, even if it seems easy to control. Any delay could have serious consequences if the fire gets out of hand. Small fires (as a general rule under $2\,m^2$) may be possible to tackle with a suitable portable extinguisher provided a clear exit is maintained.

When the fire alarm is heard it must be assumed that there *is* a fire and the building must be evacuated. Local evacuation procedures must be followed. Providing there is time, any apparatus that could cause extra problems should be switched off and all doors (and windows if there are any) should be closed.

Staff should proceed to the designated assembly point without delay so that they can be accounted for. It is far better that personal belongings are burnt than to risk burning or asphyxiation retrieving them. Human life must come first; in most cases it is not possible to save animals. Many would have to be killed if they were released.

BIOLOGICAL HAZARDS

Laboratory animals possess a wide range of micro-organisms both inside and outside their bodies. Most of these organisms are harmless but some present a high risk of infection to people working with them. The risk is present in body fluids, tissues and waste products as well as with the whole animal and could exist in an apparently healthy animal. Diseases like this which can be passed from animal to man are called zoonoses.

Pathogenic organisms can enter the human body by inhalation, ingestion or through the skin. Suitable personal protective clothing must be worn whenever biological material is being handled to prevent entry to the body by these routes, and subsequent infection.

Practices such as pipetting by mouth should never be carried out in any type of biological or chemical work.

Some animal work involves working with animals that are intentionally infected with pathogens that present a risk to the health and safety of staff. Work of this nature is controlled by the Health and Safety at Work Act 1974 and is carried out in isolation units whose design and work practices must be in accordance with guidelines issued by the Advisory Committee for Dangerous Pathogens. These guidelines describe the measures that must be taken to prevent the pathogens that are being used infecting workers and escaping into the environment.

Disposal of biological waste

The most satisfactory method of disposing of biological waste is incineration as this will kill microbiological organisms. If incineration is not possible, material may need to be removed from the premises by specialist waste disposal companies. Small amounts of non-hazardous biological material may be disposed of into the sewerage system after maceration. Disposal of biological waste should only be done according to instruction from senior staff as waste removed by an inappropriate route could result in prosecution.

Several people may have to handle waste material before it reaches its final destination. It is essential that it is packaged so that these people are protected from direct contact with the waste. Double bagging in heavy duty plastic bags, taking care not to overfill the bags, is one suitable method. The bags may be autoclaved or disinfected before leaving the unit.

Many sharp instruments are used in biological work, e.g. scalpels, hypodermic needles. Glass containers are often used and these can be easily broken giving rise to sharp pieces of glass. The risk of wounding is high and if the item is contaminated, harmful materials may be introduced directly into the blood stream. When disposing of items contaminated with biological materials it is necessary to sterilise or disinfect them to eliminate any potentially hazardous material. Sharp items (or glass containers that could easily break) must be kept separate from other waste. They should be placed in dedicated containers, e.g. a 'sharps' bin, to prevent them from causing danger to any subsequent handlers (Fig. 15.5).

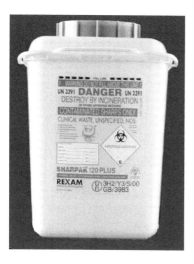

Fig. 15.5 Sharps bin.

All accidents involving work with biological agents must be reported immediately and expert advice sought.

ELECTRICAL HAZARDS

Electricity is a form of energy which can be used to provide heat, light, sound, movement etc. It consists of a flow of electrons through a conducting material (e.g. a cable). The amount of flow is called the current and is measured in units called amperes (amps, symbol A). The pressure at which the current is drawn through the conducting material is called the voltage (volts, symbol V). In the UK the standard electricity supplies are 220–240 volts. The power consumption of electrical apparatus is measured in units called watts (symbol W), watts = current × volts (W = A × V).

The amount of current that flows through a cable depends on the amount of power being used by the appliance it is connected to. Information on power consumption and current requirement should be available on the appliance itself or it can be calculated from the formula:

$$current = \frac{watts}{volts} \quad \left(A = \frac{W}{V} \right)$$

A 3 kW electric fire would draw a current of:

$$\frac{3000}{240} = 12.5 \, amps$$

A 100 watt light bulb would draw a current of:

$$\frac{100}{240} = 0.42 \, amps.$$

In order for a current to flow there must be a complete circuit. Normally electrons flow from the source through a connecting wire (the 'live' wire) to the appliance, then back from the appliance through the 'neutral' wire to the source. If there is a break in the wire or a fault in the appliance the current will not flow. However, if the opportunity arises, the current will flow through any other conductor, for instance if a human touches a live wire or appliance, the current will flow through the human with disastrous results.

More people are killed by electrical accidents than by any other type of injury. Electric accidents result in:

- Electric shock, where electricity flows through nerves, organs and muscles producing adverse reactions, for example a heart attack.
- Electrical burns from the heating effect of the current on tissue.
- Electrical fires caused by overheating or arching of the equipment when in contact with a fuel, e.g. paper.

Connecting wires, plugs and fuses to electrical appliances must only be done by a qualified and authorised electrician. Regular maintenance checks of portable appliances are required on an annual basis, to ensure that they are properly insulated and performing in a safe manner.

All rigid and flexible cables, plug tops, sockets and adapters are rated with the maximum current that it is safe to draw through them. When a higher current is drawn there is a danger of overheating, which can cause the insulation material to melt, increasing the risk of electrical shock and fire. Coiled extension leads usually have two current ratings stated on them, one for when they are fully extended and a lower one for when they are left partially wound. This is necessary because heat cannot dissipate efficiently if they are coiled. Sometimes it is necessary to use adapters to connect more than one plug to a socket, or to use an extension lead with a distribution board with several outlets in order to accommodate new or temporary equipment. Where these are used the total amount of current drawn by all of the appliances must not exceed the rated value of the cable and, whatever the rating of the cable, must not exceed 13 amps because that is the maximum standard wall plugs are designed to carry. Extension cables must not be used as a permanent power supply; if the need for the supply remains, extra permanent sockets should be provided.

The connecting plug of each piece of electrical equipment is fitted with a cartridge fuse (Fig. 15.6). The cartridge contains a thin wire which is de-

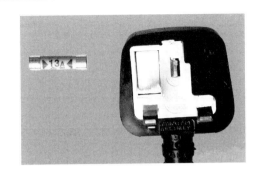

Fig. 15.6 Plug and fuse.

signed to melt (or blow) if the current drawn through it becomes too great. This will cut off the electrical supply to the appliance. Fuses are available to fit appliances drawing different amounts of current and it is important to select the fuse that will blow if the expected rating is exceeded. For instance, if an appliance should draw 2.8 amps it should be fitted with a 3 amp fuse, not a 13 amp fuse.

Any apparatus requiring a current of more than 13 A (e.g. a cage washer) is normally hard wired to its own power supply which is appropriately fused.

If there is a fault in the electrical apparatus, current may leak through the casing increasing the risk of electric shock. To reduce this risk appliances are constructed in one of two ways:

- If the appliance has a metal case it will be connected to the earth wire in the plug, the current will then flow through this wire and not the body of a person who may touch it.
- The appliance may be completely encased in a non-conducting material such as plastic which will insulate any body touching it.

Mains circuits can be constructed to minimise the risk of shock by incorporating safety devices such as earth leakage trip switches and residual current detectors which detect abnormal current flow and switch off the electric supply.

There is an increased risk when using electrical appliances in damp or wet conditions because the moisture conducts electricity over the surface of the insulating material. Dampness lowers the resistance when touching the appliance and improves the connection between an individual and earth, thus increasing the risk of injury.

To minimise the risk, electrical sockets in potentially damp areas should be fitted with waterproof covers. All electrical cables must be kept clear of small formations of puddles and a residual current device fitted, which will cut off the power source in the event of a problem. Care must be taken to prevent trailing electrical leads from becoming damaged; an example of this is allowing leads to trail over animal cages where they can be chewed, or where they can create a trip hazard.

RADIATION HAZARDS

Radiation is the term given to forms of energy propagated as waves, rays or streams of particles. Radiation is classified into two types based on the form of damage they do to tissue as they pass through. Ionising radiation (e.g. alpha particles, beta particles, gamma rays, X-rays) causes tissues to become ionised leading to cell death and severe damage to the genetic material in the nucleus. The second type of radiation is called non-ionising radiation (UV light). As the name suggests ionisation does not occur but nevertheless it can cause severe tissue damage.

Controlled radiation is used in diagnosis and therapy and it is a useful scientific tool. Both ionising (gamma radiation) and non-ionising (ultraviolet light) radiation are used as sterilising agents.

All types of radiation are potentially dangerous but provided they are used in the appropriate manner risk to those working with them can be eliminated.

Types of radiation

Radioactive materials

Radiation is produced when the nucleus of an atom is unstable and disintegrates. The type of radiation released depends on the type of disintegration that occurs; it may be alpha particles, beta particles or gamma rays.

Alpha particles – do not travel more than a few centimetres in air and cannot penetrate a sheet of paper. They will not penetrate skin; however, if they are ingested they can do a great deal of damage to tissue because they release all of the energy they carry in a small area.

Beta particles – penetrating ability differs according to the source but even the most penetrating forms can be stopped by 4 mm of glass or 1 cm of a suitable plastic material (e.g. Perspex). Beta particles have greater penetrating power than alpha particles but cause less severe ionisation.

Gamma rays – are very penetrating, requiring the equivalent of several inches of lead to absorb them. The chambers in which objects are exposed to gamma rays for sterilisation are shielded with walls of concrete 2 m thick.

X-rays

X-rays are produced when electrons hit a tungsten plate with great force. The electrons disintegrate to release heat and X-rays. The penetrating ability of X-rays depends on their energy. Those used in diagnostic work penetrate soft tissue but are absorbed by bone. Protection from diagnostic X-rays can be provided by 2 mm of lead.

Ultraviolet light sources

UV light has poor penetrating properties so it does not damage deep tissue but it does cause considerable damage to superficial tissue. The energy given up by UV light when it falls on tissue stimulates chemical reactions which can result in burns (sunburn), cataracts and skin cancers. Protection from UV light is relatively easy to achieve by covering exposed skin, wearing eye protection and using barrier creams. In each case care must be taken to ensure the material used will inhibit UV rays.

Lasers

Lasers produce a narrow beam of high intensity light that can burn tissue and cause corneal and retinal damage. Goggles and gloves must be worn and the instrument should only be used by trained operators.

The dangers of X-rays, UV light and lasers all cease when the apparatus that generates them is switched off. Alpha, beta and gamma sources emit radiation at all times and must be shielded when not in use.

General radiation safety

Work with radiation is regulated by a complex legislative framework. This controls the purchase, use and disposal of radioactive sources and the use of generated radiation (e.g. X-rays). Facilities using radiation will need to be specially designed, equipped and be frequently monitored for contamination. Staff may need to undergo regular health monitoring. Legislation requires that a qualified radiation protection officer is appointed to supervise controlled areas.

The basic principles of radiation safety can be summarised as follows:

- Keep as much distance as possible between the source and operator (the inverse square law applies: double the distance from the source and the exposure is cut to one quarter, treble the distance and the exposure is cut to one ninth).
- Limit the exposure time – radiation effects are cumulative.
- Wear protective clothing appropriate to the type of radiation in use.
- Avoid contamination, particularly ingestion of radioactive sources.
- Always wear a dosemeter (or film badge) to record the amount of exposure received.

CHEMICAL HAZARDS

All chemicals must be handled with care. Even those that are apparently harmless could react violently when they come into contact with other chemicals. Chemicals may be:

Carcinogenic Affecting cell division resulting in overgrowth of tissue causing tumours, e.g. many tarry substances, blue asbestos.

Corrosive Producing burns and other damage to tissues, e.g. strong acids and alkalis.

Explosive Releasing intense heat and large amounts of gas when exposed to a suitable stimulus such as a spark, e.g. nitro-glycerine, flour.

Flammable Catches fire easily because it has a low flash point, e.g. ether and many other solvents.

Irritant Causing local tissue reaction to their presence, e.g. dust.

Toxic Causing poisoning, e.g. mercury, strychnine, organo-phosphorus compounds.

Teratogenic Causing malformation of developing embryos/foetuses, e.g. thalidomide.

Chemicals can enter the body by the same routes as pathogenic organisms, that is by ingestion, inhalation and skin absorption. In all of these cases damage may be local or the chemical may be absorbed and distributed around the body causing a systemic effect. The amount of damage done to tissues is affected by the concentration of the chemical, the exposure time and the frequency of exposure.

Safe use of chemicals

Before chemicals can be used in a work situation a risk analysis must be carried out and measures established to ensure they are used in a controlled and safe manner (see earlier – COSHH). Hazards associated with chemicals can be acquired from data sheets supplied by the manufacturer, from information and hazard signs attached to the label on the chemical container and other sources. Once the hazards are identified means of controlling them must be developed. This will result in a standard operating procedure or safe work practice instructions which will detail how the chemical must be used in the workplace. Included in the instructions will be details of appropriate protective clothing to be worn and action to be taken in the event of accidents and spillage.

Staff using the chemical must be given adequate information and training to use it and must understand that it can only be used in the authorised way. A chemical used in an appropriate manner can have little or no risk attached to it but if it is misused or mishandled it can be very dangerous.

All safety measures introduced must be monitored on a regular basis to ensure that they are still effective; this is especially true for the use of personal protective equipment.

Spillage of chemicals

Before a chemical is used the hazards associated with it and the action to be taken in case of a spillage must be known. The basic principle for dealing with a chemical spillage is containment of spillage and introducing an appropriate method to clear and safely dispose of the chemical. This often means soaking up the liquid in an inert absorbent material and clearing into a suitable container for safe disposal (note sawdust should not be used for this purpose). To ensure an inert material is used, specialised spillage kits should be available.

Storing flammable materials

Bulk storage of flammable materials is controlled by Health and Safety Regulations. They must be stored in a suitable building, geographically separated from other buildings and isolated from sources of heat and interactive compounds.

Within an animal facility flammable materials should be stored in the following conditions:

- Quantities of no more than 50 litres including waste can be stored in any one work area.
- In a metal, flame-resistant lockable cabinet, with both the cabinet and the immediate area fitted with the appropriate warning signs.
- In a cool, dark, well-ventilated area.
- In suitable, sealed and labelled containers.
- Away from any source of ignition; this includes refrigerators that are not spark proof and any interactive compounds.

Storing poisons

The purchase, storage and use of many of the chemicals used in animal units are regulated by legislation. Any chemical classified as a non-medicinal poison under the Poisons Act 1972 and appearing on Schedule 1 of the poisons rules must be kept in a locked cupboard and records kept of its purchase and use.

The control, supply and use of controlled drugs, prescription only medicines and other therapeutic substances used on protected animals in designated premises are the responsibilities of the named veterinary surgeon.

Transporting chemicals

All chemicals must be transported in the correct manner. Gas cylinders should be moved in an upright position in a specialised transport trolley to ensure that the cylinder valve is not damaged. Winchesters must be transported within a dedicated Winchester holder, not carried by the neck of the bottle (Fig. 15.7).

Legislation exists to regulate the disposal of chemicals in order to prevent environmental

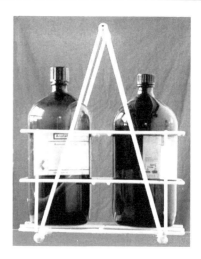

Fig. 15.7 Winchester carrier.

pollution. Highly toxic materials such as solvents must not enter sewage systems. Specialist chemical disposal companies are available to remove hazardous waste.

ACCIDENT PROCEDURES

If an accident involving trauma or unconsciousness to either man or animal is discovered it is important *not* to make things any worse! The situation should be assessed before any action is taken and, if it is possible to do so without causing danger to oneself or further danger to the injured party, the primary cause should be removed, e.g.

turn off power supply. Persons who are not qualified in first aid should then summon assistance from someone better qualified to deal with the situation.

The role of the qualified first aider is to prevent the condition from deteriorating, to preserve life and to promote recovery.

Reporting accidents and ill health at work is a legal requirement. The information can be used both at a local level and by the enforcing authorities to see where injuries, ill health and accidents are occurring, and to advise on preventive action.

Glossary

acid
substance that gives rise to hydrogen ions (H+) when in water. Reacts with bases to produce salts and water. pH < 7.

aerosol
fine mist of liquid particles in air.

alkali
substances which give rise to hydroxyl ions (OH–) when in water. pH > 7.

alloy
a mixture of metals, or of metal(s) with other substance(s), resulting in a substance with different properties.

ambient
of the surroundings.

amphibian
vertebrate animals which return to water to breed, whose immature forms live in water and have gills, e.g. frogs, toads, newts, salamanders.

anaesthesia
loss of sensation.

anaesthetic
chemical which induces a loss of sensation, can be general which also induces loss of consciousness or local which causes loss of sensation in a defined area.

analgesic
a drug which relieves pain.

ano-genital
pertaining to the anus and the sexual opening, hence ano-genital distance – degree of separation between the anus and genital opening.

arachnid
invertebrate animal with four pairs of legs, body divided into head and abdomen, e.g. spider, mites and ticks.

aspiration
steady sucking, e.g. with a syringe.

aural
pertaining to hearing.

autoclave
pressure vessel that is used for high temperature steam sterilisation.

avian
pertaining to birds.

axillae
(Singular – axilia.) The space between the upper part of the fore limb and the side wall of the chest – 'armpit'.

bacteria
very large and widespread group of microscopic, single-celled organisms. They may be free living, parasitic or saprophytic. Some are pathogenic on animals, man or plants.

cadaver
dead body, especially complete.

cantilever
projecting, rigid support.

carcase or carcass
dead body, especially dismembered.

carcinogen
agent which may cause cancer.

caustic
having corrosive properties, e.g. alkali such as caustic soda (sodium hydroxide).

-cide or cidal
agent which will kill, e.g. bacteriocide.

colony
groups of animals kept together for a particular purpose, usually breeding.

corrosive
substance that disintegrates materials, especially metals or living tissues.

crepuscular
animals active at dawn and dusk.

decipher
to unscramble, decode, turn into understandable sequence.

dermal
of the skin.

dermis	lower layers of the skin beneath the epidermis.	intractable	difficult to manage.
dessicator	large glass vessel designed for the gentle drying of crystals.	ion	electrically charged atom or group of atoms formed when a molecule dissociates (splits).
dewlap	a pouch-like fold of skin, under the chin of rabbit or on the chest of cattle.	ionise	to cause an ion to be formed, e.g. by radiation.
ecto	on the outside of the body, e.g. ectoparasite such as flea.	lagomorph	herbivorous mammals similar in structure to rodents but with an extra set of incisors, e.g. rabbit or hare.
endo	within the body, e.g. endoparasite such as a tapeworm, endodermis – inner lining.	larva	developmental stage of invertebrate, e.g. maggot.
epi	above, or outermost, e.g. epidermis – the outermost lining.	litter	young animals born to a mother at one time.
excreta	waste materials from the body, especially urine and faeces.	litter	bedding material, or under cage 'bedding' material, or material provided simply to absorb urine and cover faeces.
flammable	susceptible to combustion.		
gait	way of walking or running.	lux	unit of light intensity.
genitalia	the primary sex organs. External genitalia refers to the penis and scrotum of the male or the vulva of the female.	mammal	endothermic vertebrate, with hair, that bears live young which it suckles.
genital papillae	rudimentary, developing genitalia.	mammary gland	organ which produces milk.
genetic engineering	artificial techniques used to alter the genetic make-up of an organism.	meatus	a passage such as the ear canal (external auditory meatus).
haemorrhage	escape of blood from a vessel.	metabolism	chemical reactions that occur within an organism.
hock	joint in the hind legs of animals that corresponds to the tarsal joint or ankle.	metabolic rate	rate of metabolism, e.g. use of energy.
homeostasis	maintenance of a constant internal environment in an animal's body.	mite	microscopic free-living or parasitic arachnid.
		molars	back teeth used for crushing and grinding.
hyper	over, e.g. hypersensitivity – increased sensitivity	mucous	secreting mucus.
hypo	under, e.g. hypodermic – under the skin.	mucus viscous	(thick), sticky or slimy fluid secreted by cells.
inbred	offspring produced by mating close relatives.	nocternal	active at night.
		nymph	immature form resembling adult.
incisors	front 'biting' teeth.	occlude	to block or obstruct.
inert	chemically or physiologically inactive.	ovum	female sex cell or gamete, egg.
		oxidation	combining with oxygen.
insect	invertebrate animal with body divided into head, thorax and abdomen, three pairs of legs on thorax, often with two pairs of wings, e.g. ant, bee, moth, flea, louse.	palpate	to feel gently with the fingers.
		parasite	organism living on or in another organism (its host) and obtaining its food from it.
		Pasteurella	group of bacteria causing diseases

	such as plague, septicaemia, pseudo-tuberculosis.
pathogen	organism capable of causing disease.
peninsular	protruding like an island.
penis	erectile sexual organ of male used to introduce sperm into vagina of female.
pH	numerical scale indicating degree of acidity/alkalinity.
pinna	ear flap.
posture	way of holding the body.
prolapse	slipping out of place of an organ, e.g. prolapsed rectum – a rectum protruding through the anus.
protein	complex organic compound made of amino acids, required for producing body tissues and compounds such as hormones, enzymes and antibodies.
puberty	process of change leading to sexual maturity.
pupa	developmental stage of some insects, e.g. chrysalis.
quarantine	isolation from others in order to prevent the spread of infection.
rectum	last part of the intestine opening through the anus.
reptile	four legged vertebrate animal with dry, horny skin. Many lay eggs with leathery shells, others bear live young, e.g. lizards, snakes, turtles.
rodent	gnawing mammal with pair of large, permanently growing incisors in upper and lower jaws, e.g. mice, rats, hamsters, squirrels.
Salmonella	a group of bacteria causing e.g. typhoid, food poisoning – Salmonellosis.
scrotum (scrotal sac)	pouch of skin into which the testes of most mammals descend at puberty.

sentient	conscious, responsive to stimuli.
scruff	loose skin at back of neck. To scruff – hold by same.
sibling	offspring from the same parents.
spermatozoon	a sperm, motile male sex cell or gamete. (Plural spermatozoa.)
-stat or static	prevent multiplication, e.g. bacteriostat.
sterile	free from living organisms.
sterile	incapable of reproduction.
teat	nipple through which milk passes from the mammary gland.
testicle (testis)	male reproductive organ producing spermatozoa in fluid and male hormone testosterone. (Plural testes.)
toxic	poisonous.
ubiquitous	found everywhere.
vagina	duct connecting uterus to vulva, receives the penis of the male during copulation.
vapour	gas formed from a liquid.
vector	carrier of disease.
vermin	unwanted, objectionable animals.
vertebrate	animal with a brain enclosed in a skull and a spinal cord enclosed in a vertebral column.
virus	disease-causing particles incapable of multiplying outside of living tissue. Individual particles are too small to be seen with a light microscope.
visual display unit (VDU)	screen of computer, television etc.
vitamin	organic substance which, though necessary only in small quantities, plays a vital role in metabolism and is essential to support normal health.
vulva	external parts of the female genitalia.
weaned	not dependent on milk.

Appendix 1

Table A.1 Summary of the breeding of laboratory animals.

Species	Mating season in controlled conditions	Type of Oestrous Cycle — Duration of oestrus	Mechanism of ovulation	Time between oestruses in the unmated animal	Age at first mating	Gestation period	Average litter size weaned	Age at weaning	Recurrence of oestrus	Average litter interval or no. of litters/year	Average expected productivity per female	Duration of economic breeding life
Syrian Hamster	no definite season (more variable in winter)	*polyoestrous (continuous)* usually an evening	spontaneous	4 days	6 weeks or paired at weaning	16 days	6	21 days	post-partum then end of lactation	7 weeks	nearly 1/week	6 litters 8 months
Mouse (outbred)	no seasonal variation	*polyoestrous (continuous)* usually an evening	spontaneous	4 or 5 days	6 weeks	20 days	8	19–21 days	post-partum then end of lactation	4.5 weeks	nearly 2/week	6 litters 6 months
Rat (outbred)	no seasonal variation	*polyoestrous (continuous)* half a day	spontaneous	5 days	F 10 weeks M 12 weeks	21 days	10	3 weeks	post-partum then end of lactation	6–7 weeks	1.5–2/week	6 litters 8 months
Guinea Pig (outbred)	no seasonal variation	*polyoestrous (continuous)* 1 day	spontaneous	15 days	F 3 months M 4 months	about 9 wks	3.5	2 weeks (180 g–200 g)	post-partum then end of lactation	4 litters/yr	14/year	8 litters 2–3 years
Rabbit	no definite season (more variable in winter)	*governed by induced ovulation* weeks if not mated	induced by mating		Dutch F 6m M 8m NZW F 8m M 10m	28 days 31 days	7	5–8 weeks	post-partum then about 4th week of lactation	4–5 litters/yr	32/year	10–12 litters 2–3 years
Ferret	February to July	*seasonally governed by induced ovulation* weeks if not mated	induced by mating		F 9 months M 12 months	6 weeks	8	6–8 weeks	end of lactation or next season	just under 2 litters/yr	14/year	probably 6–8 litters over several years depending on condition and performance
Cat	no definite season but some variation	*polyoestrous (sometimes irregular)* 7–10 days if not mated	induced by mating	about 3 weeks	F 9 months M 12 months	9 weeks	4	6–8 weeks	about 4th week of lactation	just over 2 litters/yr	10/year	
Dog	no definite season but some fluctuation	*polyoestrous (very long cycle)[1]* about 5 days	spontaneous	6–7 months	F 12–15m (second oestrus) M 18 months	9 weeks	4	6–8 weeks	6–7 months (regular cycle)	2 litters/yr	just under 7/year	

[1] Often regarded as seasonally monoestrous.

Index